The Treason Within

The Threat To Your Health, and How To Combat It

Dr. John Millward B.M., B.Ch.

"A nation can survive its fools and even the ambitious. But it cannot survive treason from within."

Cicero (106-43BC)

Dedication

I wish to dedicate this book to my wife Vicky. She was the first person to introduce me to the opportunities offered by complementary medical treatments. In recent years she has encouraged me to write this book, which has occupied both our thoughts during the past three years.

I am very grateful for the help and training offered to me by:-

Dr. David Spence and his colleagues at the Bristol Homoeopathic Hospital.

Professor George Lewith, Dr Julian Kenyon and Dr. David Dowson who practised at the Centre For The Study of Complementary Medicine in Southampton.

Dr.Fritz Schellander – The Liongate Clinic, 8 Chilston Road, Tunbridge Wells.

The late Dr. Helmet Schimmel of Baden Baden.

And last but not least, Chris Woollams for his invaluable advice, support, and knowledge that made possible the publication of this book.

Important notice

The author is a fully qualified health practitioner, a doctor of medicine. However, the contents of this book, in part or in total, are not intended as an alternative to specialist advice for any individual disease, or any individual's illness. Each individual and their particular illness can vary and so specialist advice should be sought for accurate diagnosis and before any course of treatment.

The author and publisher cannot be held responsible for any action, or lack of action, that is taken by any reader as a result of information contained within the text of this book. Such action is taken entirely at the reader's own risk.

Whilst the author has made every effort to ensure that the facts, information and conclusions are accurate and as up to date as possible at the time of publication, the author and publisher assume no responsibility.

First published in August 2005 by:
Health Issues Ltd.
The Elms, Radclive Road, Gawcott, Buckingham, MK18 4JB
Tel: 01280 815166
Fax: 01280 824655
E-mail: enquires@iconmag.co.uk

Cover design by Jeremy Baker

ISBN 09542968-6-9

Printed in Great Britain by Bath Press Ltd, Lower Bristol Road, Bath BA2 3BL

About the author

The author was born in Brierley Hill and moved to Dudley when eighteen months old. After attending Dudley Grammar School he did his National Service serving with the Royal Artillery in the Canal Zone, and was lucky enough to travel to Sinai, Petra, Maan, Amman, Jerash, Jerusalem and Bethlehem. He went to Oxford to read Chemistry, but decided instead to read Medicine. After qualifying he worked at St. Bartholomew's Hospital and the Women's Hospital Wolverhampton, and after a short time in General Practice in Wolverhampton moved to Bournemouth.

At Bournemouth he worked in the same Practice for many years, and become involved in the local community, even serving as a Councillor on both Dorset and Bournemouth Councils. Slowly becoming concerned at the rapidly increasing workload and the inability of medicine to halt this rise in illness he began to question his position within mainstream medicine. The practice seemed to have a large number of patients, both male and female, who had developed cancer. Despite expressing his concerns he was reassured that there was no real increase in the number of patients affected by this disease. We all now know that he was wrongly advised and that he was witnessing the early signs of the present cancer epidemic. He had also taken part in various drug trials and became increasingly aware of some of the unfortunate side effects that complicate the use of drugs. Curiosity led him to watch a homoeopath at work and was surprised at the success of the treatment of a patient that had defied the best endeavours of a consultant dermatologist. Stimulated by this experience he studied homoeopathy at the Homoeopathic Hospital in Bristol and later at Southampton. He increasingly used homoeopathy and acupuncture in the NHS practice and found that more and more patients preferred these forms of treatment. Eventually he plucked up courage and left the N.H.S to set up an Alternative Medical Practice with his wife Vicky. He has studied with a variety of English and Continental specialists and increased the range and variety of his alternative medical skills. The practice has gone from strength to strength and now welcomes patients from all over the United Kingdom and abroad. He spends more time lecturing on various subjects including many of the topics found within this book. He is anxious to ensure that as many people as possible can enjoy the knowledge that offers the prospect of good health in an age that has witnessed a rapid increase in all types of acute and chronic ill health. In an effort to put back into the NHS something in return for all that the service gave to him he served for eight years as a non-executive director of the local hospital.

Foreword

I obtained my medical degree following years of study at Oxford University and St. Bartholomew's Hospital in London. To complete the course I also needed to obtain a B.A. degree in animal physiology. However my original intention had been to obtain an Oxford chemistry degree, and so my school years had been devoted to the study of mathematics, physics and chemistry.

Those formative years spent studying the physical sciences were both a blessing and a curse when I eventually came to apply my medical training to the treatment of my patients. I quickly realised patients didn't conform to any rigid scientific formula. The uniqueness of every human being, both in mind and body, can lead to an equally individual response to medical treatment. With hindsight I am amazed that I was unprepared for this eventuality. Even more amazing still is that the medical schools still teach rigid models of disease, their pharmaceutical treatment, and the further drug treatments to counter the side effects of the originally chosen drugs. The newly qualified doctors are left to discover for themselves that the practice of medicine is as much an art as a science.

My training could have led me into a career in the pharmaceutical industry, because of the belief at that time in the infallibility of science in general and chemistry in particular. A second curse came with the discovery that products of the chemical industry could have such diverse, unforeseen and often harmful effects upon the very patients that they were designed to help. After many painful experiences I came to realise that I was not as open-minded nor as questioning, as I had been led to expect would be the natural outcome of my years of training.

The treadmill of medical practice became faster and faster and with it came the realisation that there was a constant increase in all forms of chronic illness which defied all attempts by conventional western medicine to influence the outcome. My own practice became particularly concerned because we felt that the incidence of cancer was reaching epidemic proportions. As a result of enquiries we were reassured that our particular practice was unusual and that countrywide there was no significant

ix

increase in that disease. How sad to realise now that our own experiences were a true reflection of the health of the whole country, and that so much time had been lost. I am both sad and angry that I spent so many wasted years in the pursuit of improvement in health care for my patients whilst using drugs that could never provide the results that I craved. As the book proceeds you will discover not only how simple the origins of disease are but how simple safe and effective are the means of achieving both prevention and treatment. It will be for you the reader to decide if the failures of current health care are due to accident or deliberate intent.

So I was forced to embark upon what has proved to be an exciting voyage of discovery into other ways of diagnosing and treating patients. My journey has unearthed a wealth of knowledge in a variety of treatments that range from the ultra modern, based on very scientific principles, to those therapies and treatments that are thousands of years old. As more and more people come to share this knowledge it is likely that many people will turn their backs to the present day traditional western medicine, whose future looks increasingly bleak and bankrupt. Close scrutiny of western traditional medicine based upon synthetic pharmaceutical products reveals that any potential benefits may be outweighed by the consequent damage that they can cause. This situation has been compounded by the pollution of our environment by the manufacture of so many chemical products.

This book is designed to offer you the reader a choice of many different ways in order to achieve good health. There are many challenges to all those with enquiring minds. I never intended this to be a vast medical textbook that of necessity would rely upon the work of many different authors. Relying upon others risks the repetition of incorrect data. It is often said that any mistakes that appear in a medical textbook may take up to 50 years to be removed. Therefore, in the following pages you will find **my own** current views upon health, prevention and cure. However, you will find many references to other authors, books, audiotapes, factual data etc that in turn could lead you upon your own unique voyage of discovery. I hope that you can look forward to a voyage of discovery that is as exciting as mine has been. If this book is instrumental in launching you on such a voyage then the purpose of writing it will have been achieved. Day by day more and more exciting new information becomes available. This tempts me to continually rewrite and update the contents of this book. However, to do so would mean that the book would never be completed. Therefore, I have decided that no new information will be included after August 2005. I do, however, hope that you will rise to this challenge and add your own postscripts so that the voyage of discovery will continue for many more years but with different hands at the tiller.

You may find the contents of this book disturbing when you discover just how unimportant your health is to those people we trust to influence and govern our society. At times, animals appear to receive better health care than people because of their commercial value. However it may appear surprising that the health of so many people is so callously compromised by relatively few powerful people. All sections of society have elements of corruption, and the controllers of health care are no exception. Hence my choice of title for this book is **The Treason Within.**

If you are impatient and wish to discover the cause and treatment of some illnesses that affect you, your family or friends, then I would suggest that you proceed to Part 2 and Chapter 13, and read the earlier chapters later.

Contents

Appendices

PART 1

The Treason Within

"An enemy at the gates is less formidable, for he is known and carries the banners openly. But the traitor moves among those within the gates freely, his sly whispers rustling through all the alleys, heard in the very halls of government itself. For the traitor appears not as a traitor; he speaks in accents familiar to his victims, and he wears their face and their argurments, and he appeals to the baseness that lies deep in the hearts of all men. He rots the soul of a nation, he works secretly and unknown in the night to undermine the pillars of the city; he infects the body politic so that it can no longer resist. A murder is less to be feared."

Cicero (106 to 43BC)

Chapter 1

The Disaster We Should Have Avoided

There can be no doubt that modern allopathic medicine is failing us. The hopes and aspirations recorded at the start of the twentieth century were misplaced; the result, a massive increase in **all forms** of chronic disease. Medical and pharmaceutical establishments proudly boasted that they could improve upon, or even replace, the thousands of years of evolution and our naturally acquired immunity. Statistically we may live longer, however any statistical gains in longevity have been paid for by a massive increase in all forms of chronic disease (The World Health Organisation has stated this on more than one occasion). Many of these conditions were unknown or unrecognised as recently as the 1940s and 1950s. Despite this, the medical establishment still clings to the belief that in time "something will turn up" to reverse the tide of ill health.

In a recent newspaper article a professor, engaged in cancer research, is reputed to have claimed that the scourge of cancer was in the main due to cigarette smoking, overexposure to sunlight and promiscuous sexual habits. One might have expected him to offer some advice on the obvious lifestyle changes that could cut down the rate of cancer. Instead, there was the proud boast that in 50 years time there would be a cure for cancer. Perhaps someone should have mentioned that present cancer rates for men are 1 in 2 and for women 1 in 3. Projections suggest that there will be a 100 per cent cancer rate long before the 50 years have elapsed. Will there be enough people unaffected to administer the prospective cure? Present indications are that the number of ill people will very soon outstrip the capacity of the medical and allied professions to cope with their workloads. The increase in demand for hospital treatment is running at around 10 per cent per year, yet the increase in money available either seems to assume no increase in patient demand, or that the money goes elsewhere within the health economy.

How could we have allowed such a disaster to occur, or worse,

3

its very existence to be denied? There are still members of the medical profession who insist that the current heavy workload is but a tribute to their own improved skills and techniques. Furthermore, they claim that these diseases have always existed and that only in recent years have the diagnoses been made. Such views may be of comfort to doctors but not to patients. Yet the greatly increased rates of death from cancer and heart disease are not disputed. Politicians and others in positions of power and influence, and who are encouraged to commit even greater financial resources to the health services, have either been unwilling to acknowledge the failures, or that an accepted increase in illness forms part of their long-term strategy for our future.

Foolishness, ignorance and greed have all contributed to the decline in health. In the heady years of the 1950s and 1960s we all chose to forget the lessons of history. For thousands of years the human race has always struggled to survive. The fittest have survived and there has been a continuous process of evolution to adapt to the continually changing environment. However the pace of change in our environment during recent years has been far greater than anything previously experienced, and has thus outpaced the abilities of natural evolution. So we chose to turn our backs upon history and instead placed our faith in science (or rather science fiction) and the supposed superiority of mankind. Since the fateful decision was made to place our trust in allopathic medicine there have been countless battles 'fought for the good of our health' and, almost without exception, they have been lost.

In Chapter 3 there will be a description of one such defeat that occurred in the summer of 1962. Only a small group of doctors and their families were aware of this particular tragedy, and its full significance was not immediately recognised. Perhaps those struggles were far too one-sided, because some corporations, including the pharmaceutical, tobacco and petrochemical industries, were well established and possessed both the financial muscle and access to the ears of successive governments. Successive defeats have led to an even greater dependency upon those same industrial corporations, rather than to a major review of the strategy for health.

4

In any conventional war successive defeats would result in the replacement of the generals and even to the fall of governments. However, despite the fact that the war against disease is almost lost, many people still put their faith in the same generals and politicians. Unfortunately, many corporations and individuals grow rich as a result of the continuing ill health of countless people. The new NHS plan talks of putting patients first and also offering choice. Although the reality of these two concepts remains unclear, it is obvious that there is significant resistance to any form of treatment other than the allopathic pharmacological approach to disease. Many patients no longer accept the present orthodox approach without question. Such resistance to ortho-dox treatment should be encouraged, and an open, fair and ratio-nal debate on all treatments instituted in the very near future. The morale of the medical profession is at an all time low. This is due in part to an unbearable work load, and in part due to the knowl-edge that an increasing number of patients are losing faith in their practitioners and are no longer prepared to accept without ques-tion the diagnoses and treatments that are on offer. As this book unfolds, you the reader will be faced with a variety of choices. Will you dismiss its contents as foolish scare mongering and continue to put your faith in established modern medicine? Or will you choose to take greater responsibility for your own and your family's health? You may even be brave enough to help fight the battles and to win the war for that most precious gift of good health as a result.

For the benefit of younger readers it is pertinent to describe the realities of medical practice 40 years ago. General practice then was certainly less hectic than the present workload of family doctors. GPs were then referred to as family doctors, a term that reflected the patient's opinion of a doctor, who not only knew the family but was also respected for their knowledge and honesty. Patients were invariably seen on the same day that they requested to be seen. Appointment systems were the exception rather than the rule and it was a case of first come first seen. Despite this open access surgeries invariably finished on time, and not all the time was taken up with consultations. There was no fixed, short time allocated to each patient. There was ample time for home visits and during most of the year there was plenty of free time during the day to relax with the family or to perform other personal tasks. Life became more hectic during epidemics. Night visits were also rare events. I can remember visiting every old age pensioner once every month and in the summer months finding the demands upon my time almost non-existent. I am sure no one will need reminding of the realities a visit to a GPs surgery today.

Hospitals were equally relaxed. Medical patients could occupy hospital beds for weeks or even months. Of course, times could be hectic but I cannot remember patients lying on trolleys for many hours, nor can I remember having difficulty in finding hospital beds. However, within a few years of leaving hospital employment I can remember the winter epidemics causing shortages of free hospital beds. This led to the introduction of special administration units designed to hunt for available free hospital beds and thus allowing GPs to deal with other patients.

Chemists' shops were also very different. There were very few antibiotics, sleeping tablets and tranquillisers available and because of the limited choice and need they were kept in very large containers. The few cough linctuses and antacids were similarly kept in large glass containers. In fact, the whole stock could be kept on two or three shelves. At about the same time the pharmaceutical companies commenced a monthly publication, called mims, which listed all the proprietary medicines. At that time it consisted of a very few sheets of folded A4 paper. Today the monthly publication is a square ended volume of over 400 pages. This demonstrates the veritable explosion in the number of patented medicines. When you next have cause to visit your GP you will likely see a copy of mims on the desk, close to your doctor.

What did the future hold for newly qualified doctors in 1960? For hospital doctors there was a very long wait before becoming a consultant. In some of the more popular specialities the chances of promotion to consultant rank were very slim indeed. Today there has been an explosion in the number of consultants. There is currently growing pressure to even double the numbers of consultants to try to cope with the ever-increasing demands placed upon the healthcare system. Another complication has arisen following the introduction of a European regulation that limits the number of hours that doctors can work. The junior hospital doctors have traditionally worked for very long hours, and the introduction of these regulations has created an instant shortage of available qualified doctors. It is claimed that this lack of clinical experience will inevitably result in poorly trained consultants. To overcome this problem, one suggestion has been to reduce the years spent in medical training so that new consultants can be available much earlier. There is a tendency for even greater specialisation. This has lead to pressure for even yet more consultants to cover these new specialities in the event of illness, off duty and holidays. Increased specialisation has its own hazards, with fewer doctors willing to undertake routine work. Patients may request explanations for their symptoms that are outside the terms of reference of that speciality but are usually met with the comment that it is not in that consultant's sphere of knowledge. Invariably, that is where matters rest and the patient remains confused and in doubt. I remember working with a gynaecologist who hadn't examined a male patient for many years and was confused, and even embarrassed, when having to examine a male friend who had been taken ill and there were no other doctors available.

For the entrant into General Practice during the 1960s the future was even less certain. I have already explained that at times there was insufficient work to totally occupy the time of such doctors. New and exciting drugs were being introduced almost on a daily basis. There was cortisone, the wonder drug that was expected to alleviate asthma, eczema, arthritis and many other conditions. There were other new medicines for the treatment of arthritis and high blood pressure. The oral contraceptive pill was introduced and this opened up all sorts of possibilities for family planning and a possible reduction in demand for obstetric and gynaecological services. We now know that the demand for gynaecological hormone prescriptions, consultations and operations has increased rather than decreased. The many new antibiotics appeared to offer a future free of drug resistant bacteria. Today there are frequent reports of 'super bugs' that cause death and serious illness. There were very few indications at that time of the serious side effects of medicines that were to appear in later years. Was it therefore surprising that many young doctors like myself wondered if we would become redundant before becoming established in practice? Many went abroad to find countries with fewer doctors than here in England. Countries like Australia and Canada welcomed them with open arms. How unfounded were those fears when viewed from today's world of overworked doctors and an expanded training programme to satisfy the need for yet more doctors to cope with the greater demands for medical care?

In the early 1960s there were social changes that affected the status of general practitioners. Previously the cleric and the doctor had equal status within society. With an increase in the fragmentation of family units, increased urbanisation and greater time pressures upon individuals, the role of the cleric decreased and at the same time the position of the doctor within society increased. The doctor not only offered the confidentiality of the confessional but also the therapeutic salvation to cure all ills and put to right all the consequences of living in the 'swinging sixties'. Thus the concept of the infallibility of medicine was born. There are large numbers of people who continue to believe that this remains true.

In the 1960s the doctors basked in the glory of their newly found social status. However, sole responsibility is fine when all is well. When things go wrong there is no one else to share the blame. Today, doctors have to shoulder their responsibilities and despite attempts to blame the politicians and others, the buck appears to stop with them. The blame for the great increase in chronic disease must lie with them. Have they become part of the conspiracy to perpetuate illness, or are they themselves a victim of that same conspiracy? Throughout their career from student days until retirement, the giant drug companies control, either directly or indirectly, their medical education. With increasing workloads and reduced free time, doctors have come to rely more and more upon the drug companies to keep them up to date with newer developments. It is therefore possible to argue that doctors are more sinned against than they are themselves sinners. However, they are guilty of not having sufficiently independent and personal opinions. Many doctors continue to ignore the failings of a system, which readily accepts the numerous and often fatal results of using drugs. Recent research in the USA has found that properly prescribed, properly taken medicines were the 4th largest cause of death in that country.

Chapter 2

Undue Influence By Drug Companies Upon Training Of Doctors.

Doctors have to serve the potentially conflicting interests of both patients and the drug industry. What do we expect from our doctors? Of course we expect to receive treatment for any illness that we may develop. We expect to be seen promptly, and that any treatment we receive should be both safe and effective. Is that all that we should expect?

The word doctor means teacher, an additional role to that of healer. That is a role that sadly has been neglected. They should advise upon keeping well and how to avoid illness. We should expect to receive either the individual opinion of a doctor, or at least the collective wisdom of the various national bodies that represent the whole medical profession. There are many national and international issues that could have a profound effect upon the health of all of us. Many of these issues will be referred to in this or later chapters. However requests for advice are usually greeted with stony silence. It is interesting to note that the various churches are re-entering this void and expressing a collective view upon major problems that could impinge upon the social fabric of society, and also having views upon issues affecting health. In the spring of 2001 the church had forthright views upon the effects of Foot and Mouth disease. Government heeded these views. Little or nothing was heard from the medical profession. Perhaps this is an early indication that the social role of the doctor is declining while that of the church is increasing? In defence of the medical profession it is worth noting that the Labour Government chose to ignore the views on GM foods as expressed in the British Medical Journal.

The doctor's role as a teacher has been sadly omitted from the medical curriculum. This is equally true of both undergraduate and postgraduate training. The art of communication has also been omitted from medical education. As a result there are many subjects that are either omitted from the various courses or dealt with in a very superficial manner. Doctors may qualify without spending a single day learning about nutrition and body energy, both of which are essential for the understanding of disease and their role in healing. There is a requirement for ongoing training after qualification but this is essentially treatment-based. As a result there are many topics in which doctors lack the knowledge and skill with which to answer the various questions posed by patients. Such lack of knowledge even extends to the cause of many of today's illnesses. As a result of this lack of knowledge many doctors resort to a variety of techniques to cover up this vacuum in their medical education. Sadly these ruses are failing to impress an increasing number of disgruntled patients. In later chapters I will describe how many of the diagnoses are both worthless and meaningless. A medical diagnosis nowadays is only a tool to assist in the search for the correct drug, and does not identify the original underlying cause of the patient's illness.

It takes many thousands of pounds to train a doctor. So why has the money not been put to a better use? On entry into a medical school the students are told that they are joining an elite force and that their present skills of observation will be further enhanced. In addition, throughout their training, they are never encouraged to cultivate an open mind. Yet despite these noble ideals it appears that from a very early stage in their training, every effort is made to discourage open-minded thinking and the powers of observation strictly restricted to certain defined areas. When I trained to be a doctor students were continually told that the ancient treatments, including acupuncture, homoeopathy, aromatherapy, reflexology and many others, were forms of quackery that were, at best, useless and, at worst dangerous. Students were warned that flirting with such unorthodox treatments could lead to suspension from the medical register. I was taught that even discussing such treatments with a patient could lead to a similar fate. No wonder very few students or qualified doctors have strayed from the perceived orthodox wisdom. It certainly delayed and inhibited my interest in the study into the various alternative therapies. There was some easing of this official attitude when acupuncture was demonstrated to be effective but it was felt that only qualified doctors should practise it. There has however, been no rush to train them. A study comparing chiropractic treatment with conventional therapies demonstrated its superior benefits, yet once again there has been no rush to embrace chiropractics within the NHS. There has been no increase in the length of training for medical students, and so all the increased medical knowledge that has been acquired in recent years has been crammed into the syllabus with some of the basic skills squeezed out.

Nearly all training for medical students revolves around the principle that the use of pharmaceutical products is the right, proper and only way to treat patients. Side effects of medical drugs are accepted as the norm. We are constantly told that any disadvantages are outweighed by potential benefits. However, if there is only the slightest hint that a non-prescription alternative treatment could have a possible side effect, there is immediate and widespread condemnation. It is believed that a homoeopathic treatment has never been a cause of death, but as we will see in a later chapter it is a common occurrence with pharmaceutical products.

Before seeing their first patient, students receive teaching in the use of medicines. Even today, students are still taught that for a specific medical condition the drug of choice is product A. That the side effects of drug A can be countered for by the use of drug B. Thereafter drug C can be used to alleviate the effects of drug B. This perceived wisdom appears to be accepted without any question. **Yet it should be remembered that nearly all medicines suppress the symptoms of disease and neither treat nor cure the underlying pathology.** Therefore patients may be condemned to a lifetime of medication, with all its consequent side effects, so that the manufacturers can continue to earn money at the expense of both the unhealthy patient and the taxpayer.

Why should this happen? It is a matter of record that many teaching hospitals throughout the world are dependent upon financial contributions from multinational conglomerates, usually the pharmaceutical companies. Governments' contributions are also to a certain extent influenced by the desire to maintain a financially healthy drug industry. These same drug companies heavily fund medical research in medical schools, universities hospitals and many independent laboratories. It is not unknown for either individuals or organisations to have their funding withdrawn if they depart from the defined line or come up with results detrimental to the drug companies' own financial interests. Many medical charities and other organisations receive money from these same companies that have their own vested interests.

The influence of the drug companies is felt in many other areas. There are free publications aimed at the various sections of the medical profession. These publications carry many advertisements and for many hard working doctors the articles contained within these pages constitute the **only** medical reading that they have time for. Drug companies also sponsor the majority of post-graduate meetings and conferences. Some doctors also receive financial help with their travel expenses. A significant proportion of members on the various regulatory bodies own shares in the drug companies whose very products they are paid to pass judgement upon. Their ownership of these shares is declared but doesn't invariably preclude them from taking part in a debate or voting upon the final approvals. This situation is frequently highlighted in the national press, most recently concerning the licensing of vaccines, but it doesn't result in a government response or even widespread public anger. This conflict of interest would not be allowed under the code of conduct adopted by all public and most private organisations. In marked contrast, regulation of alternative health products is both rigorous and often obstructive. Decisions by officials can often be at an individual's whim in the knowledge that such actions are unlikely to provoke the wrath of their superiors. In the USA members of the government, the civil service and the professional medical bodies leave their current positions to take paid employment with drug companies. There is also a flow of people in the opposite direction. It is therefore impossible to recognise who is the gamekeeper and who the poacher. It has been reported that in January 2003 the FDA was so short staffed that it was offered 500 staff by the drug companies.

Chapter 3

Summer of 1962:
Does Good News Get Suppressed?

In 1962 I failed to appreciate how preventing the availability a single drug would come to have such a profound effect upon the health of countless millions of people. Instead my fond memories of the summer of 1962 are of long, hot and sunny days. Perhaps this was nature's way of compensating us for the long cold winter that was to follow. In January of that year I had joined a practice in the industrial Midlands. It was in an area that I was familiar with because it was near to the hospital in which I had worked, and so it offered me the opportunity to pursue my interests in obstetrics, gynaecology and paediatrics. There were three existing partners, and I was an assistant with a view to becoming a partner in the forthcoming August or September.

Most of our patients were away on holiday. The car industry, at that time, was the major employer and the employees who were directly or indirectly employed in this industry were all sent on holiday simultaneously. This phenomenon was known in all the seaside resorts as the Birmingham fortnight, when the predominant tongue was that of the Black Country accent. With so little work to do, it was an ideal time to reflect upon the past few months and to assess the future. During the early part of the year there had been a measles epidemic. It was the first of at least three epidemics that I have experienced during my medical career. I have therefore seen a large number of children suffering from this viral illness. However, I cannot relate my experiences to the picture of dire consequences as painted by the proponents of the MMR vaccine program. Perhaps it was, as the anti-vaccine lobby suggests, a disease naturally becoming less virulent. It is argued that with the passage of time the population builds up a significant degree of immunity and that the symptoms of illness become less and less severe. This theory argues that with the passage of time the childhood illnesses that we know would have slowly

14

disappeared. If this theory is right, then the unfortunate consequence of the present immunisation program is that in time those not immunised, and even those immunised against a similar but not identical virus, would lose their natural immunity and suffer far greater symptoms when faced with a genuine major epidemic. However, very few of today's family doctors have ever seen a case of measles, are less likely to make an accurate diagnosis, and have been caught up in the hysteria that has been generated by the medical/pharmaceutical establishments and then exaggerated by the media.

The measles epidemic of 1962 had meant a large number of house calls on alternate Mondays for almost two months. There was also the usual influenza epidemic. Despite this I still went home at a reasonable hour having completed my home visiting list and conducted an open access surgery. There were no outstanding surgery appointments left over for the next day and, as yet, the concept of booking appointments had not materialised. Despite the fact that this was the "busy period" there was still free time during the day and, as mentioned elsewhere, all the patients over 65 years of age were visited before the end of the first week of every month. Night visits were rare and the last visit would usually coincide with the playing of the National Anthem on television. I doubt that today's family doctors would recognise such an existence, as they contemplate various forms of protest against their exceptionally onerous workloads

The most senior of the three doctors in the practice was chronically ill, and it was to help with this situation that I had been employed. Despite the fact that this partner was unable to do his full share of the practice work, we had still managed to cope in the way described in the previous paragraph. However it was the future of the second partner that most excited me. He had an interest in diseases of the chest, and had worked part time in the local hospital. He had also been involved in a research project with a major pharmaceutical company. The company was about to bring to the market a new drug that would be capable of killing all viruses. It was not recognised that the success of such a drug could damage the future prosperity of drug companies by reducing the amount of chronic illness and a consequent reduction in the demand for drugs. This new medicine was to have the same effect upon society as Fleming's discovery of penicillin. It was pointed out to me that this would eradicate colds, influenza, measles, mumps, chicken pox and many other viral illnesses. In turn this would reduce the amount of work time lost through illness and would have a profound effect upon the national economy. In our practice this would leave only chronic back pain as the sole major cause preventing patients attending for work. This dramatic advance in medicine, combined with the introduction of such wonder drugs as cortisone, reinforced my view that many doctors would be redundant and that it would be more difficult to obtain a job in general practice. Indeed as mentioned elsewhere the contraceptive pill had also just reached the market, and it was assumed that this might in turn lead to a reduction in the number of doctors required specialising in obstetrics and gynaecology.

With so much uncertainty facing the future employment prospects of doctors, I was delighted to be offered a partnership. It was not intended that I should become a fourth partner, but I was to replace the middle partner who would be leaving to take up a full time career in the hospital to pioneer the introduction of the new anti-viral drug. It was envisaged that after a short interval of time the project would go nation-wide. It was easy to visualise that three partners, even if one of them was unfit to practice full time, could easily cope with winter pressures especially when this new drug became available. Unfortunately at the very last minute, at the very time we were due to sign contracts, the drug company withdrew from the project without, as far as I am aware, giving any explanation for its decision. In the local community only the four practice doctors and their families knew of both the project and its cancellation. The second partner was to remain in the practice, and he and his two colleagues were prepared to honour their offer of a partnership. For a variety of reasons I felt unable to stay, and after being unemployed for several weeks found a vacancy in a practice in Bournemouth. With the financial pressure of unemployment and then a new practice I temporarily forgot the loss of yet another wonder drug.

On Boxing Day 1962 the snow reached Bournemouth and

stayed around for many weeks. Bournemouth was unprepared for such an eventuality. Getting about and visiting patients was a nightmare. Many patients were without water because water pipes that had been laid too near the surface and consequently froze solid. We soon came to recognise and treat hypothermia. The hospitals gained experience in coping with multiple fractures. I gained insight into the various ways in which a viral illness could present, because the isolation of many families ensured that I could be certain that the same virus was responsible for any febrile illness that occurred within a family.

In the following years viruses appeared to have an even greater effect upon medical practice. Everyone was told that they had a virus. Patients accepted this sort of diagnosis and antibiotics were freely prescribed even though there was no evidence that their use was of any benefit. In later years patients accepted that antibiotics were of no use and therefore were happy not to have them prescribed. Sometimes the diagnosis was more specific, as in the case of glandular fever, even though this was originally thought to be a hysterical manifestation. Later diagnoses included post-viral syndrome and ME to name just two. There are still large numbers of doctors who believe that there is a considerable element of mental illness in such patients and this has resulted in the widespread use of various anti-depressant drugs.

Today my mind travels back to 1962, and I now wonder why that specific drug was withdrawn at the very last minute. I do not remember any financial statement being made nor that shareholders in the company witnessed a drop in the value of their investments. Today such a withdrawal would be headlines in the financial press, and there would have to be a statement to the shareholders and the Stock Exchange. In parallel situations today there might be an investigation and a possible fraud trial (a recent trial alleged that a doctor's trials of a new drug that had led to a consequent rise in share price had been shown to be at best inaccurate). As the years have gone by there have been many new powerful drugs that have found their way onto the market. During that time one or two expensive products have been introduced for certain specific viral diseases. The results of using these drugs are not reliable nor without undue complications. Is it thus

17

impossible to manufacture an anti-viral compound? Patients are repeatedly told that there isn't an anti-viral drug, except for the specific examples mentioned above. How is it that there are several specific anti-viral homoeopathic preparations available? These preparations are cheap to produce, they are free from potentially harmful side effects, and are totally effective in both acute and chronic viral infections.

So why are these specific homoeopathic remedies not in general use? Is it because they cannot be patented and are therefore of no financial benefit to a drug company? So we must once again look back to 1962. It is very doubtful that the drug was too toxic to be introduced onto the market. It is equally doubtful that had there been any toxic problem it couldn't have been rectified during the past forty years. If this anti-viral drug could have had such a profound effect upon the nation's economy, why didn't the government intervene with advice, help and financial support?

An alternative explanation could be very damaging to the reputation of drug companies. There have been examples where patents have been bought out to prevent a rival's product reaching the market place where it would compete with the buyers' own products and thus damaging that company's prosperity. Of course, there is an alternative hypothesis for the 1962 decision to withdraw the prospective anti-viral drug. Let us assume that a decision was made on financial and not clinical/chemical grounds. Could it be that the company realised that the reduction in viral illness could drastically reduce the demands for the company's other products? Worse still, is it possible that other companies were consulted and reinforced that particular financial view? Could there have been a conspiracy involving many companies? The reality is that there is now a demand for more and more drugs to suppress the symptoms of long-term, and sometimes viral, chronic illness. There has been a switch to multiple vaccination programs in an attempt to prevent viral diseases. This demand for vaccines is a long-term money-spinner. If, as seems likely, there were adverse consequences resulting from these injections that in turn would require further medicines to suppress the unwanted symptoms, then this in turn could lead to even greater income to the companies. It is a win-win situation for the drug companies even if it is at the expense of the poor unfortunate patient.

Everybody agrees that there has been a progressive and unrelenting increase in the workload of doctors. A significant proportion of this increase has been attributed, rightly or wrongly, to both the acute and chronic effects of viral diseases. These viral diseases have caused profound suffering in very many patients. Prescription medicines rarely bring relief and more commonly lead to unpleasant side effects. **It is unbelievable that no plausible treatments for viral illnesses have existed for at least 40 years. In the unlikely event that these potential medicines were either ineffective or too toxic, why has the medical establishment in the UK refused to embrace the use of those particular resonance homoeopathic remedies that have proved to be effective? We are left with a conspiracy theory that ill health, and its consequences, is too important for the wealth creation of certain powerful people and their associated organisations, and therefore anything that might improve health must be resisted.**

Chapter 4

The Death Of The NHS?

"As to diseases, make a habit of two things – to help or,
at least, do no harm"
(Hippocrates)

Only drastic action can save the health care system. A complete change of direction is required. I have already mentioned the increased workload experienced by all doctors working within the National Health Service. The solution offered by doctors is for more government money to include the funding of a large increase in the numbers of new doctors, nurses and other paramedical specialists. It is painfully obvious that a significant proportion of the increased workload is due to their own drug-based approach to medical treatment, and consequently their salvation is in their own hands. Eventually the increasing spiral of work and associated cost will be broken either by patient pressure for change, or by a bold government that reduces the funding of the Service and yet demands better treatment and an associated fall in the level of illness. However at present the almost daily publication of medical health scandals in papers, periodicals, on radio and on TV hasn't as yet excited enough people to force any governments to act. I believe that any legislation would have to be embraced by all governments because large countries like the USA would claim unfair restriction of trade if the products of their multinational companies were banned or controlled from entering other countries.

General Practitioners have always prided themselves in their independent status, and their role as a gateway to the whole of the healthcare system outside and beyond their own practices. A system of medical ethics is still in place that prevents full and free access to the system other than with the consent of the General Practitioner. This is an outdated practice that should be discontinued. Abolition of this practice of referral is in the interests of both patient and doctor. As the pressure builds up within any system, the time will come when the force of pent up energy will break down the barriers and overwhelm those areas beyond the obstruction. General Practice will disintegrate and the doctors will take all the blame. At a recent conference of the British Medical Association the following comments were attributed to its Chairman: "His members were being made scapegoats for a system in crisis". He demanded "an end to doctor baiting and doctor bashing". "We have become scapegoats for the failings of a system with grossly unrealistic expectations, whipping boys when Government can't live up to its manifesto pledges, victims of a complaints culture fuelled by the hysteria surrounding medical mistakes". His verdict on the Government's record during the preceding four years: "Four years on, our hope has turned to despair and disenchantment, our saviours have become our accusers and our morale has been driven to distressingly new depths".

As you read this book you can decide for yourself if doctors themselves are to blame, or if others are equally culpable. The Government will distance itself from catastrophe and join in the condemnation of the whole medical profession. Is this a remote possibility? I doubt it because the medical press (the free newspapers funded by the drug industry) is already reporting an increasing number of physical and verbal attacks upon doctors. Doctors themselves are lamenting the fact that an increasing number of patients are failing to show them the respect that they feel they deserve. If any more proof is needed, consider the fact that the cost of litigation against both doctors and hospitals is increasing at an alarming rate The cost of litigation against hospitals, which is borne by the NHS, and ultimately the taxpayer, is causing politicians a great deal of concern. Doctors working outside hospitals have to provide their own insurance. These premiums have also risen and for 'safe' procedures amount to 6 per cent of income. Poor communication between health professionals is frequently the root cause of complaints that proceed to litigation. However rather than addressing the basic causes, doctors are inclined to bemoan the fact that there are other and better ways in which money spent upon litigation could be spent on direct patient care.

With the deterioration in the relationships between doctors and their patients, it is worth studying the methods of communication employed by doctors. The crowded curriculum for medical students has already been mentioned, and thus it can be no surprise that little attention is paid to the teaching of communication skills. Dr. Stewart Mercer, who is disabled, made four comments on what he learned from his own handicap. Two of his comments are very relevant in this context. They were: "Good medicine is more than technical skills and knowledge", and: "An ability to listen, empathise and communicate are core skills for doctors".

The 'bedside manner' may be inherited, acquired during the working life, or in many instances never learnt. The methods of communication have changed little in the past 50 years. The only real difference is the very blunt manner in which the terminally ill patient is told about the diagnosis, treatment and likely outcome. Other diagnoses are meaningless. A diagnosis of Irritable Bowel Syndrome (IBS) is a classical example. It means "that there is something wrong with your bowels and that it is affecting the quality of your life. We have carried out several investigations but have found no obvious cause". Then why not admit that something is happening but you don't know what? There is usually a cause to be found, one which will I will explain in later chapters. However the outcome for the patient is a variety of different medicines, which are designed to relieve symptoms but not to eradicate the underlying cause. Stress is hinted at as a possible precipitating factor, but at least the patient is spared the indignity of being labelled a neurotic. It seems that even the diagnosis of stress is frequently misplaced in that there is usually some hidden pathology that causes the symptoms. The diagnosis of stress represents the personal view of the doctor, it may have been a spur of the moment judgement, but this particular diagnosis is incapable of confirmation by routine medical investigation. One magazine claimed that lazy doctors were to blame for the large increase in morbidity and time off from work that was associated with labelling patients as suffering from stress. However stress is a word that patients feel comfortable with because everyone knows of other people that have been given the same diagnosis.

22

The use of the word stress is becoming a social and financial problem for the patient, the employer and the national economy. The Government is concerned at the high rates of sickness absence from work, and has commented that stress is a major cause for concern. In the absence of any firm diagnosis the patient is left to his or her own devices and spends months or even years searching for the least upsetting diet and possibly consulting one or more alternative practitioners.

There are other chronic conditions like ME (chronic fatigue, post-viral syndrome) and fibromyalgia that medicine has had difficulty in coming to terms with. At one stage even the now well-recognised glandular fever was viewed as a mental condition. These chronic conditions often defy all attempts at proving that there is a single infective cause responsible for each individually named disease, and this leads to the suspicion that there is a significant degree of mental illness rather than any physical pathology. It is therefore no accident that various anti-depressant drugs are routinely prescribed. To satisfy the flawed medical logic that there should be a single cause for each illness, a Dorset hospital studied patients with ME, and failed to find evidence that one specific virus was present in all these patients. The inevitable result of this research led many physicians to believe that ME was a psychological problem rather than a physical illness. At least a proportion of doctors now accept that these illnesses do occur. However sceptical doctors, when faced with the prospect that alternative medicine has been successful, will argue that it is wrong to give the patient the false impression that they had a physical problem rather than their real mental problem This concept that a patient's belief in a physical cause for their illness is erroneous is at best offensive to the intelligence of both the patient and alternative practitioner. The word alternative here applies to anyone using anything other than allopathic medicines, and thus depriving the pharmaceutical companies of ongoing income.

Prior to the introduction of current pharmaceutical medicine, doctors had to rely upon their knowledge of both the patient and the family plus the power of their own personality. Any failure on the part of the patient to get well was attributed to the lack of any real effort on the part of the patient. Thus the doctor's reputation was preserved at the expense of the patient's self-esteem. This attitude still persists today. Doctors often misunderstand many of the symptoms that are of real concern to patients. Many patients are greeted with, " what do you expect at your time of life", or, " it's normal for a woman of your age", or, "I am also tired and depressed", or "its still a virus". Age, stress and hormones are the favourite diagnoses. In recent weeks I have come across two unusual comments. A General Practitioner confronted by a woman of 68 years who had no discernible major illness that he could find is reported to have said, "you have only got four or five years left. Do you really want something doing?" Another gentleman consulted his doctor because of hay fever and other allergic symptoms. He enquired about allergy testing and any possible alternative treatments to the ones he had already tried. He was told that, "all allergy testing and treatments were a waste of time, were quackery". Furthermore he was also told that if he really wanted to get rid of his allergies "he should go and live on the moon".

So where do doctors stand today? Certainly overworked, relatively unsuccessful in treating chronic illness and feeling paranoid that patients and politicians are all plotting against them. One false move could result in litigation, therefore the temptation for a doctor to refer the patient to yet another doctor. In reality what is the state of the health in our so-called affluent society?

Fifty years ago parents were concerned for their children because of the threat of nuclear war. Few people at that time were concerned about the effects of radioactive leakages from nuclear power stations and other nuclear establishments. Today's parents are more concerned about cancer affecting members of their family. This fear is justified with cancer rates soaring to affect about one in three people, with men being afflicted more than women. Despite extensive and expensive treatments for cancer the cure rates remains stubbornly poor. Heart disease, which is also increasing, doesn't have the same glamour and publicity as cancer but is still currently the number one killer, although likely to be soon overtaken by cancer. Quite obviously these two diseases have occupied the attention of doctors, politicians and statisticians. However as the World Health Organisation has noted, other chronic illnesses have also increased in incidence and probably mirror the rise shown for cancer and heart disease. These changes in all chronic diseases are demanding upon doctors' time, and are becoming increasingly expensive to treat. The only people to benefit are the shareholders of the pharmaceutical companies. More work, more time coping with illness, more morbidity and the result is a health care system itself in terminal decline.

In later chapters I will argue that at least four out of every five cancers are preventable, and that the one in five people that develop cancer could be treated more successfully and humanely than at present. The same reasoning applies to heart disease and other chronic illnesses. If the numbers suffering from these illnesses are so well known, why don't doctors inform patients and give them the option of trying different therapies? Why don't they educate patients or more importantly stand up to governments and major companies when their actions are manifestly against peoples' best interests?

Patients are denied the knowledge about the rise in chronic disease and their poor record of treatment. In the United States of America it is officially estimated that medical practice in general is the third most common cause of death. The various medical causes responsible for deaths of 225,000 people in one year are shown below.

Unnecessary surgery	12,000
Medication errors in hospital	7,000
Miscellaneous errors in hospital	20,000
Infections in hospitals	80,000
Non-error, negative effects of drugs	106,000

The figures for deaths due to medicines could be stated in a simpler fashion by saying that for every person who died because they were given the **wrong** drug, fifteen others died as a result of being given the **right** drug!

It is estimated that 40,000 UK citizens every year may suffer a similar fate. In February 2003, the national press carried articles citing the publication of official estimates that 800 babies "are killed every year by poor NHS care", and that "53 per cent of these infant deaths were as a result of avoidable error".

If, as claimed, four out of every five cases cancer and heart disease are preventable, then this could catapult death due to medical practice to the number one spot in the list of causes of death. Thus either by omission to practice preventative medicine or 'malpractice', places doctors in a very precarious position. The question arises as to why they continue to allow this state of affairs to persist?

The present British Government, so obsessed with data collection, must be in possession of the necessary information to enable it to publish the estimated annual deaths attributable to medical errors. It does propose to introduce a new system of reporting of what it calls adverse health care events and near misses. It intends to draw upon the experiences of both the United States of America, and of Australia (another country with a poor record of medically induced deaths) before finalising its plans. However in the UK it has stated that:

- Approximately 85,000 adverse events take place a year (roughly 10 per cent of hospital admissions).
- Adverse events cost approximately £2 billion a year in additional hospital stays.
- 400 people die, or are seriously injured, in adverse events involving medical devices every year.
- Every year the NHS pays out around £400 million in settlement of clinical negligence claims.
- Hospital-acquired infections, around 15 per cent of which may be avoidable, cost the NHS nearly £1 billion every year. (In an earlier report the Government claimed that about 5,500 people die from hospital-acquired infection every year. The Government now publishes a league table of hospital cleanliness. In an apparently odd quirk of statistics it has found that some of the cleanest hospitals have a higher rates of infection).
- Adverse events cost approximately £2 billion a year in additional hospital stays.
- Around 1,150 people who have been in recent contact with mental health services commit suicide every year.

It is obviously much easier to note and report adverse events that occur within the hospital environment rather than in the wider community. However the Government has set out various targets that it expects the health service to achieve and these include:

- To reduce by 40 per cent the number of serious errors in the use of prescribed drugs by the end of 2005. (This would appear to exclude the recording of death or serious disability as a result of prescribing the correct drug. It can be seen from the previous text that the number of deaths due to the correctly prescribed drugs exceeds the deaths due to incorrectly prescribed drugs by 15 to 1).
- To reduce to **zero** the number of suicides by mental health patients as a result of hanging from non-collapsible beds or shower curtain rails on wards by March 2002. (I cannot verify that this target was met).

These two targets, and the others, seem difficult to achieve as long as governments continue to yield to the financial pressures of the pharmaceutical companies and to deny patients the alternative treatments that appear both safer and effective.

Most damaging is the conclusion that doctors appear to have betrayed the trusts of millions of people who have been brought up to regard their profession as being there to serve in the best interests of patients. Many people still instinctively believe in their doctors' integrity, but should we now reassess this view? Are they the real villains, or are they too the victims of a conspiracy by other more powerful groups of people? The Government has been tempted to specify certain recommended treatments for some specified individual diagnoses. This would further deny doctors of any individual opinions, and could even increase the number of unwanted adverse events. Are doctors therefore willing or unwilling architects for the inevitable decline in the health of populations?

Chapter 5

Tobacco And Cancer:
The Economics Of Illness

Cancer is claiming the lives of countless people. The death toll from this potentially preventable disease is increasing at a frightening pace. If you live in a democracy you are entitled to expect that the elected government will act on your behalf, to give you protection, and value for the money in taxes collected from you. It also has to balance the interests of the other contributors of taxes, including industry. A healthy environment is a basic human right and an individual should expect to have good food to eat, clean water to drink and pure clean air to breathe. Unfortunately most people are denied these basic rights. Cancer Research UK claims that in the year 2000 there were 270,000 new cases of cancer, a 40 per cent increase in 25 years.

You should expect to be served by a well-educated and capable civil service that services and advises an administration containing honest and well-qualified politicians. In addition any government can call upon the services of leading academics and also the leaders of commerce and industry. In recent years a series of events have caused concern and called into question the reliability of the advice and actions of government. More and more people are discovering that they can no longer accept without question the advice offered by the various ministries. Information that is freely available to everyone appears to be discounted and ignored. With more people questioning government policies the whole credibility of democratic government is called into question. There has been a blurring of the edges between the truth, 'spin' and lies.

In this book we are concerned only with health issues. The media is taking a very keen interest in this topic, presumably reflecting the public's general concern. However in most cases the issues are only highlighted but seldom ruthlessly pursued. The first and vital question is why any government would continue to

28

increase funding into a state healthcare system with diminishing returns? Illness is increasing as outlined in previous chapters, more people are joining the long queues for medical attention and the service is just begging for evermore increasing amounts of money to recruit more staff and open more hospital beds. Despite this the media continues to highlight the shortcomings of what it describes as a 'Third World' service, but contributes little to the debate on how to radically influence our health. The staff working within the NHS complains of overwork but appear unable to appreciate the true reasons for the crisis. Why are there no demonstrations and calls for action by, or for dismissal of the government? The political parties in opposition in Parliament appears equally unconcerned by the situation, only offering advice on how to spend more or less money within the present system. Surely someone should ask the **present Government** to explain why there are more ill people nowadays.

Perhaps the demands for greater investment in the NHS should be resisted until a fraud and waste figure of between £7 billion and £10 billion (identified below), which represents between 16 per cent and 20 per cent of the total funding, has been addressed. The Governments own statistics include:

- £2 billion lost because of 'adverse events' e.g. bed blocking (the patients who are fit medically, but remain in hospital because of the failure to make alternative arrangements for their future care. The agencies responsible for finding suitable alternative care for these patients are themselves starved of government funding.)
- £ 1 billion to £3 billion lost through fraud such as patients falsely claiming free prescriptions and dentists charging for treatment not carried out.
- £2 billion on sick pay and agency nurses. Back injury accounts for about 40 per cent of this and may be due to incorrect lifting of patients. A recent private industry report claims that 15 per cent of illness is not genuine. Perhaps this is why the Government has made the reduction of sickness one of its targets. Traditionally public sector services have a poor record when dealing with sickness absence.

- £1 billion to treat hospital-acquired infection.
- £300 million to £600 million through over-prescription of drugs.
- £400 million on clinical negligence claims by patients.
- £230 million treating patients who become malnourished.
- £150 million on avoidable health and safety measures for staff.

Since the end of the Second World War many people have been apprehensive about the adverse effects of nuclear technologies used for both civilian and military uses. Official reassurances have done little to dampen people's fears. Leakage of nuclear products still happens and clusters of various cancers occur in certain parts of the country. In recent months there have been various press reports of military personnel being used as guinea pigs both at sites of nuclear test explosions and at Porton Down. After the Gulf War there occurred a variety of serious illnesses amongst servicemen. Rather surprisingly there has been reluctance on the part of Governments to consider the possibility that these diseases could be the result of modern nuclear tipped weapons or from the various measures, like the use of vaccines, taken to combat the effects of exposure to chemical and biological warfare agents. These are some of the examples of the unwillingness of governments to listen to the concerns of affected people and to resist all forms of independent enquiry.

However the longest, and possibly the best-known saga concerns the relationship between tobacco and cancer. Chewing tobacco has long since been known to cause cancers in and around the mouth. 40 years ago very strong evidence was produced linking smoking and cancer. The first identified link was between smoking and cancer of the bronchus. The evidence was so strong that many doctors, especially those involved in chest surgery, turned their backs upon smoking and turned instead to the whiskey bottle. A group of doctors recently wrote to the Lancet urging governments to ban all tobacco products. Over the years the evidence of the harmful effects due to smoking have been verified time and time again. Other cancers, including those affecting the bladder, have also been linked to smoking, as has heart disease, the other leading cause of death in the western

30

democracies. Women appear to be at twice the risk of developing cancer. Despite this young women appear to have developed the tobacco addiction. Passive smoking has also been identified as a potent cause of cancer and many other diseases. It is estimated that nine out of ten people who are exposed to other people's cigarette smoke are as much at risk of developing diseases as the smokers themselves. Despite the mass of evidence, and the pressure upon Governments to take action, very little has happened. To their credit doctors themselves have led attempts to persuade politicians to take a firm stand. Perhaps the Government does realise that reducing smoking would lead to a reduction in cancer, but refuses to take action against the tobacco industry because it would then be forced to acknowledge and tackle the many other industrial causes of cancer. Perhaps governments place a greater emphasis upon the tax revenues that they raise from these companies rather than the health of the population. Governments may feel that the loss of tax revenues due to the banning of tobacco would cause a major financial crisis and also an increase in unemployment. In the UK the tax revenue from tobacco is estimated to be around £2 billion daily.

The only enforced significant changes have been the addition of health warnings on the packets plus the information of tar content. Now there are plans to remove some of the many toxic additives. The companies have raised no significant objections and therefore we can assume that they had already decided to do it. In a token effort to reduce the numbers of smokers nicotine patches and a new product called Zyban have been introduced into the list of products authorised for use by the National Health Service. Nicotine is addictive and therefore continues the dependence and also there is ample evidence that it can react with other ingredients in tobacco smoke to form carcinogenic compounds. The dangers of the nicotine therapy have been documented both in the professional literature and in the national media. So far the present Government has not acted. Zyban has been linked to several unexpected deaths that have received extensive publicity, and doctors too have expressed their concerns regarding the use of this drug. However the medical profession is under pressure from the Government to reduce the numbers of deaths due to heart disease and cancer. Unless smokers can be persuaded by their doctors to cease smoking without the use of any medication it seems likely that doctors will be damned if they prescribe and damned if they do not. Therefore the Government is relying upon the medical profession to curtail the smoking habit, preferring not to legislate against the tobacco firms. There is a silver lining for the drug companies who now have yet another income stream from the treatment of those diseases that result from the smoking of tobacco. The court cases in America against the tobacco companies rely upon the fact that those companies knew that their products caused cancer but failed to tell the people.

There has been no significant legislation to protect non-smokers from the effects of inhaling other people's tobacco smoke. Many restaurants and licensed establishments have to cope with the conflicting interests of smokers and non-smokers. There have been several recent comments that the Government might consider banning smoking in public places. Despite this, an attempt by the European Union to ban smoking in public places was opposed by the British Government. Instead of legislation to ban smoking in the workplace, the Government appears to be relying upon the various restaurants to take the initiative and to run the risk of losing customers. It could also be relying upon the trade unions that are becoming more proactive in the protection of their members from the effects of passive smoking whilst at work in restaurants and licensed premises. Several local authorities are considering bye laws to introduce such bans, however without government support such bans are deemed to voluntary and unenforceable. Despite pre-election pledges to curtail tobacco advertising, the Government failed to act until mid-February 2003 when it introduced a partial advertising ban in certain public places. However there have been exceptions to this ban, notably formula 1 motor racing. No attempt has been made to deter the aggressive promotion of cigarette smoking in many of the Third World Countries where levels of disease are already far too high. Perhaps it is perceived that the financial health of the tobacco firms is more important than the physical health of the people of those countries targeted for the expansion of cigarette sales.

The above comments should come as no surprise to the reader. The following is but a small selection of headlines that have appeared in both the lay and professional papers. "How passive smoking can cause asthma". "Passive smoking can kill your cat". "One puff a day can damage your heart". "How a single cigarette can hook a child". "Three cigarettes a day can double a woman's risk of a heart attack". "Cancer threat from second hand smoke beyond doubt". "Cancer will kill 5 million British smokers". "Nicotine patches 'danger'". "But passive smoking can undo the good". "Researchers raise fear over long-term nicotine therapy". "Zyban makers ordered to be at girl's inquest". "Is nicotine a tumour risk?".

There has however been one particularly chilling newspaper headline: "Tobacco firm says smoking deaths boost economy". This particular article was remarkable because no other paper appeared to have taken up the story, nor has there been any response from any government. The newspaper itself failed to produce a follow-up article. The story related to the alleged comments made by an adviser to the tobacco manufacturer Philip Morris. This had been in response to a statement that smoking was a drain upon the financial resources of the Czech Republic. The adviser argued that cigarettes save the economy millions in **health care because smokers die early.** It was argued that savings on **health care** and **pensions** far outweighed the cost of looking after smokers who fall ill with cancer and heart disease. The savings to the Czech economy were estimated to be £100 million annually. The calculations included the income from excise duty and healthcare costs savings due to early death. Savings still accrued despite decreased tax revenue from the deceased or ill smokers.

Should this single newspaper report be taken seriously? I believe that it should be, and that the lack of further articles and especially the absence of official comment, are both highly significant. Were these comments too near to the truth for comfort? Was it assumed that this lack of comment would lead to the early loss of interest in this subject? For every article printed on the subject of smoking related diseases there have been many more articles on the perceived failures of the health care system. There

33

have been significantly fewer articles on the marked increase in all forms of illness, from whatever cause, and there appears to be no attempt to associate this increase in disease with the failure of the system. More alarming is the fact that there seems to be little account taken of this increase in illness when planning for the future needs of the NHS. There are however very many articles written about the crisis in pension provision. The Government has acknowledged this concern over pensions. There is talk of delaying the age at which pension is paid and that longevity and early retirement are partly to blame for the pension crisis. Companies are trying to decrease their pension provisions and everyone is encouraged to take out private pensions and to continue working for extra years. So there seems more than adequate reason to take the Czech report very seriously. What applies in that country could equally apply to this and other countries. Could this in part explain why successive governments have failed to take action against the tobacco companies? Could this also explain the lack of government action against the pharmaceutical industry despite its failure to halt disease and the obvious harmful side effects of their products? Is this also why the American government persists with its vaccination policy despite having to pick up the costs of early adverse and acute reactions to the procedures?

Tobacco is only one of many products, including medicines that are potentially harmful to health. Other examples appear in later chapters. Thus there is a major political dilemma. The tobacco, petrochemical and pharmaceutical industries employ millions of people and have millions of shareholders. Mobile phones and the mobile phone masts seem to pose the latest threat to health, including causing cancer. Did the present Labour Government know this when it issued licenses in return for very large fees? Would any move against the various products that are harmful to health trigger a stock market collapse and therefore massive unemployment? If the decline in health continues at the present rate then that too will threaten to reduce the available workforce. Industry needs workers and governments need tax income from employees' salaries. Delay will not make decisions any easier.

Chapter 6

50 Years Of Avoidable Dangers
To Your Health

During the second half of the twentieth century several major industries have blossomed, and despite safety concerns, successive governments have encouraged their continued growth.

The history of the nuclear industry is relatively short, but ever since the explosion of the first nuclear bomb there have been concerns about the effects of radiation upon human health. Despite concerns, the industry has expanded to include power generation, medical uses, and reprocessing, in addition to the various military applications.

The immediate and long-term effects of the bombs dropped on Japan are well documented. However 50 years after the post war nuclear tests held in the Pacific, there are repeated claims of ill health experienced by the many servicemen who were present at those tests. Governments have resolutely opposed the claims. However produce grown in areas surrounding the test sites would appear to be still contaminated with radioactive residues. During recent military conflicts depleted uranium shells have been fired. It is claimed that the use of these shells poses no risk to military personnel. However despite this there are many claims of ill health arising from their use. Again both the American and British Governments have tended to dismiss these claims. The officials sent to the battlefields where these shells had been deployed claim to have found evidence of excessive radiation. Yet Governments have also dismissed the Gulf War syndrome as a myth. However the picture has been clouded by the use of multiple vaccines and chemical cocktails to protect soldiers against the possible use of biological and chemical weapons. Servicemen spent hours in armoured vehicles that magnified the already high levels of electromagnetic radiation from computers, radios and other electrical equipment. The need to combat dehydration required increased fluid intake and with it the chemical aspartame, a known toxic chemical, and a common ingredient in low calorie drinks. Following years of sustained pressure it is likely that Governments may yield and institute various enquiries. However, any enquiry that starts with the premise that vaccines depleted uranium and aspartame are safe is unlikely to be fruitful. Several recent enquiries have added to this suspicion in that by setting deliberate terms of reference any government can ensure that it escapes blame. Despite the official denials of a link between the cocktail of inoculations and the Gulf War syndrome, a recent War Pensions Appeals Tribunal hearing has awarded a soldier a war pension on the grounds that these vaccines damaged his health. It will be seen in a later chapter that any vaccine is capable of causing unsuspected illness. The more vaccines and fillers that are in any given injection, the greater the chance of unwanted side effects.

Nuclear power has always had its critics. These concerns are far wider than the two major accidents, the one in America and the other at Chernobyl. The Russian explosion demonstrates just how far the radiation can spread and affect populations thousands of miles from the site of the accident. Welsh lambs were declared unfit for human consumption because of the fall out of pollution that contaminated the fields and water where these animals had been kept. Workers at nuclear plants, their relatives and those other people living near to these establishments have frequently expressed concern over the possible health dangers associated with these organisations. Clusters of various types of cancer victims have been recorded as living, or have lived, near to these plants. The authorities have accepted that a few of these cases have resulted from exposure to radiation. There appears to have been several accidental radioactive leaks, some airborne, others waterborne. Nuclear facilities are supposed to monitor their immediate environment to detect evidence of leakage, but reports of such events seldom become public. The French reprocessing plant on the Cherbourg peninsular has conducted a great deal of research into waterborne pollution and how it spreads. They are more reticent about their own monitoring of any airborne pollution and the publishing of their findings. However although the French authorities claim that there is no evidence to suggest that waterborne pollution poses any threat to human health, the scientists that work at this establishment, and who are aware of the research data, restrict the amount of shellfish that they themselves consume! Their research not only plotted the sea currents and the spread of radioactive materiel but also the degree to which various aquatic creatures and flora absorbed and retained any radioactive materiel. It is of note that the farmers on the Channel Islands use large amounts of seaweed to fertilise their fields. Radioactivity of seaweed has been measured, but has it been traced onwards into the various crops?

In January 2002 a Cornish M.P. unearthed the records of an accident involving the disposal at sea of radioactive waste. It was reported that for a period from 1965 to the early 1980s civilian and military nuclear waste was dumped at sea about 250 miles to the west of Cornwall. These operations were carried out by a variety of ships and crews with no expertise in the handling of nuclear materiel. Several accidents have been reported including one dumping where not only was the ship's position unknown but, a glass container was broken on board ship exposing both ship and crew to radiation, and that barrels containing nuclear waste were deliberately pierced so that they would sink more easily.

Medicine embraced nuclear technology for both diagnostic and therapeutic purposes. However these usages appear to have diminished as a consequence of the realisation of the dangers posed by X-rays and radioactive isotopes. The degree of safety when exposed to the various man-made pollutants (both chemical and radioactive) has been much disputed. Various national regulatory bodies determine the so-called safe limits of exposure. Many people believe that these limits are far too high. Many manufactures claim that their products are in safe low dosages and that they pose no danger to human health. So how low is safe? More importantly how safe is repeated exposure or can other environmental conditions magnify the effects of the radiation? Should we, for instance, accept the irradiation of our food when the dosages used are very high and in the face of evidence that the process damages the very cellular structure of the food?

The majority of people are aware that nuclear products can be harmful, but are less aware of the dangers posed by the products of other industries, especially the petrochemical one. The petrochemical industry produces a large number of chemicals, but very few are tested for safety by governments or other regulatory bodies. The workers in these industries may, or may not, be aware of the dangers to their health posed at their workplace by exposure to these chemicals. In 1930 1 million tonnes of chemicals were produced. Today 400 million tonnes are produced world wide. Many of these chemicals are themselves waste products formed during the manufacture of other chemicals and could represent an expensive disposal cost to a company unless some alternative use can be found. Such a solution turns a loss into a profit and therefore presents temptation to a company, which may expediently turn a blind eye to possible dangers to health. Two major examples are the use of a toxic fluoride compound to fluoridate water and dioxin-laden ash used in road building and the manufacture of breeze blocks. We are all exposed to an ever-increasing array of potentially harmful chemicals whose safety has never been tested. These chemicals can find their way into many common products that are considered to be part of normal and safe everyday life. Some chemicals that have been used in everyday life for many years have more recently been found to be harmful, but nevertheless their use is still permitted. The fact is we are exposed to many toxic chemicals that are cheap to produce, and cheaper to sell to the public rather than be safely disposed of. Researches at Lancaster University found that in testing for the presence of 78 chemicals in the bodies of volunteers, on average 27 chemicals were present.. DDT, lindane and PCBs were amongst the chemicals tested. DDT is not banned, only it's sale not permitted in the Western countries. It is available in African countries that grow fruit and vegetables for sale in the United Kingdom and therefore DDT can still enter our bodies. In 2002 a Royal commission looking into toxins in our environment found that we were exposed to 4000 substances of which the majority were toxic and that a great number were probably carcinogenic (capable of causing cancer).

Many of these harmful chemicals even find their way into prescription and over the counter medicines. When chemicals are described as being toxic it often means that they are carcinogenic. Although cancer is the major health topic, it should not be considered in isolation. Cancer is only one of many chronic illnesses that can be caused by the exposure to toxic chemicals.

American research has shown that about half of the most commonly prescribed medicines contain ingredients capable of causing cancer. These toxic chemicals can either be major therapeutic ingredients, or simply used as fillers. These claims were made either following the study of the manufacturers own data or that of government agencies. When assessing safety it appears that no account has been taken for prolonged usage, or any possible cumulative effect of mixing more than one toxic chemical. Most medicines are designed to reduce symptoms rather than to cure the underlying cause of the illness, and their inevitably prolonged usage is thus ever more likely. Chemicals themselves can change when brought into contact with the human body, and as a consequence become even more toxic. Accidental or deliberate prolonged periods of medication are very common.

Pharmaceutical companies would argue that any potential and theoretical risks are outweighed by the benefits of the medicine. However I believe that the combination of known side effects, and the prolonged usage solely designed to reduce symptoms, would counter this argument. However most patients are unable to balance the risks because they are unaware of the dangerous and toxic ingredients. Even their own doctors are not fully aware of the toxic nature of these ingredients. The manufacturers data sheets generally describe possible adverse reactions and not the toxic nature of the individual contents. Adverse effects of medicines are known to include a number of avoidable deaths caused as a result of their administration. Few doctors are likely to tell their patients that they could die as a result of taking a particular prescription medicine.

Tamoxifen is probably the most publicised example of a medicine with a sting in its tail. It is used in an attempt to prevent the occurrence, or reoccurrence, of breast cancer in those women adjudged to be at greatest risk. These particular breast cancers are either caused by, or stimulated to grow by, the patient's own oestrogen. In theory, tamoxifen and oestrogen (the former is a synthetic hormone and the latter a natural one) compete with one another at cell receptor sites. Cell receptors are very important because hormones and other chemicals influence the behaviour of cells by attaching themselves to these sites. Like a key in a lock the hormone or chemical must be of the correct shape to fit the cell receptor. The tamoxifen theory is that the patient's own oestrogen and the prescription drug each compete to fit into the cell 'lock'. The more 'locks' that are occupied by the drug then the fewer that are available for oestrogen. The patient literature that accompanies the tamoxifen tablets lists many unpleasant side effects including the fact that the drug can itself cause cancer. It is difficult to see how the benefits outweigh the risks. No effort is made to balance the argument by offering safe alternatives. "Oestrogen, the killer in our midst" by Chris Woollams, is I believe the ultimate authority on the dangers of this hormone, and is described as an essential guide for people with hormonally responsive cancers, or those who want to avoid them. "The Breast Cancer Prevention Programme" by Dr Samuel Epstein is full of practical advice on how to reduce the risk of developing breast cancer in the first place. Dr John Lee's books explain how natural progesterone is a safe alternative to synthetic proges-terone. Natural progesterone reduces the levels of oestrogen in the body. Dr Lee describes laboratory experiments in which oestrogen stimulated the growth of breast cancer cells whereas progesterone reduced the rate of their growth. Doubts about the efficacy and safety of tamoxifen are growing, but this is just a prelude to a newer generation of medicines that reduce oestrogen levels and are already being the subject of research in various hospitals. Their safety will now come under the spotlight, but it is very unlikely that they will be free from adverse effects, and therefore it seems logical to use the safer natural progesterone. The history of medicines to relieve arthritis showed that many of the newer drugs introduced following the banning on safety grounds of butazolidin, were themselves toxic, and some had to be withdrawn from use shortly after their introduction.

The moral for the medical industry is that all medicines that contain toxic, or potentially toxic ingredients should carry a recognisable warning symbol. Both the doctor and the pharmacist should draw the presence of this symbol to the attention of the patient. Failure to do so should be the subject of professional misconduct charges. What better way to start this process than by insisting that packets of HRT, the pill and any oestrogen containing medicine must contain such a warning. How can women make an informed decision unless they see such a warning and obtain further advice from doctors and pharmacists who themselves must be fully informed of the dangers. This is very unlikely to happen without massive patient protests, so in the meantime all patients must learn to question the safety of **ALL** the medicines they use. Attention also should be directed towards the non-active ingredients, especially in creams applied to the skin Patient awareness and patient power are the most important factors that will compel both government and industry to take more seriously the safety issues. It is suggested that for every toxic chemical there is always a safe and effective alternative treatment.

It is impossible to avoid all danger but it is possible to reduce the many obvious risks. Other examples of safer choices will follow in subsequent chapters.

Chapter 7

Beware!! Danger In The Home

Modern homes are full of dangers to our health. The word home should be synonymous with safety. Every parent would wish to make their home a safe haven for their children. Few parents would knowingly place their children at risk of harm, especially in their own home. Most of us were brought up to believe the kitchen to be the most dangerous room in the house, especially when hot food and liquids are about. However knowledge of the hazards posed by toxic chemicals leads to the conclusion that the bathroom might pose the biggest long-term danger to health, and therefore this room in the house becomes potentially the most dangerous. Many toxic chemicals find their way into so called 'personal care' products, which can be found in any bathroom. The term personal care can include soaps, shampoos, conditioners, hair dyes, hair sprays and gels, bubble baths, tooth paste, mouthwashes, cosmetics, deodorants, creams, lotions, scents, perfumes, various sun creams and talc. Perfumes appear to pose one of the greatest threats because there are no legal requirements to list their contents. In any perfume there may be 40 or 50 ingredients, often products from the alcohol and petrochemical industries.

The list of potentially harmful ingredients is headed by Sodium Lauryl Sulphate (an engine degreaser and garage floor cleaner) and Propylene Glycol (used as a brake fluid and de-icer). This is because they have both been used for many years, are present in many products, and because of that they are the most likely chemicals to come to the attention of anyone investigating possible harmful ingredients. They are both cheap to manufacture, and the latter creates a smooth feel while the former creates plentiful foam. Manufacturers of personal care products have attempted to divert attention away from these two chemicals by using a variety of different names in their lists of ingredients. In the list of ingredients attached to any product, the higher named chemicals are present in the greater proportions. The manufacturers of both these chemicals have to comply with strict health and safety rules. Workers wear protective clothes and any spillage and contamination is treated very seriously. The containers of both chemicals leave the factory bearing the approved dangerous chemical symbol. Extracts from the manufacturers data sheets are shown in appendix A.

A study of the list of ingredients in many personal care products will reveal that one or both of these chemicals is present to some extent. But further enquiry will reveal many other harmful ingredients are present in commonly used products. Again, examples are shown in appendix B. However for a fuller account I would recommend reading "Unreasonable Risk" by Samuel Epstein. The subtitle reads: "How to avoid cancer from cosmetics and personal care products". Although born in Scotland Professor Epstein, a world famous toxicologist now lives and works in America and is Professor of Environmental Studies in Chicago I can do no better than to quote from the back page of the book.

"Shopper beware of unreasonable risk".

According to recent daily use estimates, three personal care products are used on infants and children, ten personal care products are used by men, and women use six cosmetics and thirteen personal care products, some products are used several times daily.

Assuming mainstream industry products each contain only two carcinogens (The Royal Commission thought it could be as high as 50 per cent), this results in daily exposure to six different carcinogens for infants and children, twenty for men and thirty-eight for women.

While ingredients are listed on product labels, there is no warning as to the cancer risks from any of the ingredients.

It is unthinkable that women would knowingly inflict such exposures on their infants and children, let alone on themselves, if products routinely used were labelled with explicit warnings of cancer risks.

It is unbelievable that the powerful multibillion-dollar global

*mainstream industries continue to inflict such risks on unsus-
pecting consumers, especially as safe alternative products are
available.*

*It is equally unbelievable that regulatory agencies worldwide
still deny citizens their inalienable right-to-know of information
on avoidable cancer risks from common consumer products.*

*It is even more unbelievable that the 'charitable' American
Cancer Society and federal National Cancer Institute and 'cancer
establishments' world-wide remain recklessly silent and fail to
advise consumers, Congress and Parliaments, of scientific
evidence for these avoidable cancer risks".*

This book explains how to recognise carcinogens on product
labels, boycott such products, and shop for safe alternatives from
non-mainstream industries and thus reduce your avoidable risks
of cancer.

Professor Epstein has cited a number of chemicals that he
states can cause cancer. There are 40 'frank' carcinogens (chemicals that can cause cancer) to be found in personal care products.
There also 30 other 'hidden' carcinogens, which themselves may
not cause cancer but in certain circumstances may become
carcinogenic. Some may be contaminants in otherwise harmless
ingredients. Others can become carcinogenic when in chemical
reaction with other chemicals present. Still more can become
carcinogenic when breaking down or when in contact with skin.
Scents and perfumes contain many chemicals, some of which are
carcinogenic, but present legislation doesn't require their presence to be recorded on the label. The same requirements or rather
lack of them exist for some household cleaning products.

The FDA in America thinks it takes 9 months to look at one
ingredient. The Royal Commission said that there were 4000
such ingredients. Simple arithmetic reveals the scale of the
problem, and all the time new chemicals are being introduced
into our environment without any independent checks upon their
safety.

In addition Professor Epstein points out that underarm deodorants and antiperspirants can cause breast cancer and that the
humble talc can cause both cancer of the ovary and degenerative
lung disease. Other researchers have confirmed these findings,

and warning articles are beginning to appear in the newspapers. More examples can be found in both Professor Epstein's "Safe Shoppers Bible" and "the Unreasonable Risk", where safe alternatives are listed.

I hope that you the reader will now be sufficiently motivated to read "The Unreasonable Risk". The early pages are very readable and give an excellent summary. The rest of the book is devoted to a catalogue of safe, and unsafe, products and their ingredients. In addition to the personal care products it deals with some of the equally toxic household products, and these include washing up liquids, laundry soaps, detergents, antiseptics, glass cleaners and air fresheners. If however you find that you prefer smaller and illustrated booklets then I can recommend "Cancer-causing Chemicals in Cosmetics and Daily Use Products". It is one of a series of booklets printed by Jutaprint, Penang; ISBN 983-104-092-9.

When the use of more and more personal care products became socially acceptable and desirable, it was assumed that the skin formed a natural barrier that protected the internal organs from a hostile external environment. Today it is realised that skin is porous and may allow free passage of substances both into and out of the body. It appears that Sodium Lauryl Sulphate can make the skin even 40 per cant more porous. Medicine and the pharmaceutical industry are well aware of this and deliver medicines to the body via creams and skin patches. It was learnt that the skin was not a perfect barrier when it was noticed that there were adverse effects from products such as cortisone creams, which were intended only to treat the skin itself, but unfortunately some active ingredients entered the body causing unwanted side effects, especially in children. Despite this harsh lesson, neither doctors nor the industry has thought that it should warn people of the possible harm arising from the use of various personal care products. Some of the above toxic chemicals are even included in some proprietary medicines. Oils can block the skin pores and prevent the excretion of toxins from the body. Sodium Lauryl Sulphate as a known skin irritant is used to deliberately damage the skin of animals in order to test the effectiveness of various medicinal creams.

It is difficult to quantify the lifetime risk posed by carcinogens in personal care products. The number of products, the daily number of applications and the duration of use will all affect the outcome. Interaction between different chemicals and with the skin itself can all affect the outcome. As noted above, babies may be exposed from their date of birth and that first application of talcum powder. Women tend to use many more products than men. American research suggests that women's bodies contain about 40 per cent more toxins than their male partners. Experience with alcohol and cigarette smoke suggests that the female body is more susceptible to the effects of toxic substances. In addition there is always a person's individual response to any exposure of a given chemical.

Cancer is now an epidemic. The risks of carcinogens are there for all to see. So why take an avoidable risk? Everyone now knows that smoking causes a variety of cancers, plus other diseases of the heart, lungs and arteries. One cigarette doesn't kill you, but more than one daily over many years can do so. The same applies to personal care products, in that one application of one product on one day may be harmless, but consider the effects of using multiple products, more than once daily and over many years. Although there is more than one explanation for the cancer explosion (see later chapters), why ignore one of the commonest and vital causes?

Why have we been allowed to continue to buy and use so very many toxic chemicals that are in every day use in our homes? Industry cannot launch a new food that contains a dangerous ingredient, so why not apply the same rules to toiletries? Many of these chemicals have never been tested for safety before coming onto the market. All the information regarding the toxicity of these chemicals is freely available to governments and their various regulatory bodies. This is yet another example of how elected governments have betrayed the trust of their electors. The wealth of the very powerful petrochemical and cosmetic industries appears to take precedence over the health and welfare of people. There will come a time, in the very near future, when the damage to a population's health can no longer be ignored.

Chapter 8

The Poisoning Of Our Water

During the reign of Queen Victoria many dramatic changes occurred. The creation of proper sewerage and water treatment systems was probably the most important innovation for the improvement in the health of the nation. The Queen's own family had suffered from drinking contaminated water, typhoid contributing to the death of Prince Albert. No subsequent medical, or public, health advance has had such a significant and profound effect upon the health of this country. We have forgotten the magnitude of this advance and now take for granted the safety of our drinking water. Sadly we have forgotten the importance of simple hygiene measures. Careful observation in any public toilet will reveal that a significant number of people fail to wash their hands after using the facilities. Most people believe that if any infection arises from this lack of care, then there are always antibiotics to solve the problem. Such people could have their attention drawn to the recent article that claims no antibiotics will be effective within the next few years. Perhaps they do not realise that viruses and parasites, both common causes of stomach upsets, are uninfluenced by antibiotics. Other contaminants that can cause symptoms are not even infective agents. There are however more sinister threats to our health. The sewerage system itself is reaching the end of its useful life, and despite of repeated breakdowns there has been a lack of resources to renew it. Water treatment plants need modernisation and the final treatment and disposal of sewage itself needs massive investment. Since the privatisation of the water industry, the companies and their shareholders are anxious to limit their investment in any improvements. This is despite a massive increase in demand to satisfy our increasing dependence upon household and industrial technology in addition to the increased emphasis today placed upon personal hygiene. Doctors now place greater emphasis upon the need for all of us to drink more water, and I presume they believe that our tap water is safe. The recent problems experienced by both the rail network and the electrical supply system, each the result of neglect and under-investment, should have alerted the Government to the dangers of failing to modernise the essential utilities. No Government can fail to realise the importance of maintaining a reliable water and sewage system. If the present minor problems progress to a major disaster, either through physical collapse of the system or by the addition of toxic chemicals to water, then thousands or even millions of affected people will know that they have been compromised by the omissions of their own governments.

Are there any other threats to the safe quality of our drinking water? Firstly the increase in demand for water has necessitated that water has to be recycled many times, especially in the cities, before it escapes the system and reaches the sea. Every time that water passes through the body and back to the treatment plant there is an increased opportunity to pick up contaminants. Although water has always been at risk from contact with untreated water or contamination by sewage, there are more modern forms of pollution that require different treatment techniques. These newer techniques will require massive investment.

Bacterial infections such as typhoid may have been common in Victorian times, but today viruses and other organisms are a greater cause for concern. Many of these organisms cannot be treated by conventional medicines and are therefore free to escape from the body in urine and faeces. They may also find their way to contaminate water in the hand basin, bath, shower or washing machine. A variety of parasites can find their way into the water system. This threat is largely ignored because as will be explained in a later chapter the incidence of parasitic disease is grossly underestimated. Doctors have often been warned that what they fail to look for they will never find.

Any pharmaceutical drug used in medicine can escape from the body to contaminate water. In recent years many different chemicals have been manufactured and incorporated into our lifestyles. Many of these chemicals haven't been tested for potential toxicity before being used, but are nevertheless now known to be toxic. Meat may contain antibiotics, cortisones and other hormones. Not surprisingly these chemicals can find their way into other foods like milk, cream, butter, cheese and eggs. Chickens and eggs are well-recognised sources of food poisoning. These infections due to contaminated food may be the result of the indiscriminate use of antibiotics in farming leading to resistant organisms, or to poor farming or processing techniques.

In food processing, colourants and preservatives may be added to increase its aesthetic appeal and to extend its shelf life. Fruit and vegetables are likely to contain herbicides and pesticides plus artificial fertilisers. Fish and other marine animals that may enter our food chain will have absorbed many of the pollutants that we have dumped into the sea. This includes radioactive waste, untreated sewage and a variety of industrial waste products. Some industrial waste materiel can mimic oestrogen and has been found to have a feminising effect upon certain males in a variety of fish and marine animals. This poses a threat to the procreation and survival of certain species, including human beings.

In a previous chapter mention is made of the many toxic and cancer-causing chemicals that are ingredients in many commonly used personal care, cosmetic and household products. It is obvious that these chemicals will eventually find their way into wastewater. The many harmful ingredients found in prescription medicines will also find their way into the waste water system via urine and faeces. Some of the oestrogen that can be found in both oral contraceptives and HRT will also escape from the body. This may account in part for the reduced fertility of men and the symptoms of excess oestrogen levels in women. It is now a matter of record that the chemicals in oral contraceptives and HRT can cause cancer and when these chemicals escape into the water system they pose a cancer threat to all who drink water. Today all medicines come with a list of possible adverse effects, but fail to mention the dangers caused by their escape into the sewerage system.

In certain parts of the country, untreated water is taken from a variety of sources, including wells. These sources are increasingly prone to contamination from modern farming methods. This includes slurry, artificial fertilisers (especially nitrates and phosphates), pesticides and herbicides. Two recent reports have linked nitrates with some cancers of the oesophagus, and the European

Union has criticised the UK for having drinking water containing nitrates in excess of the recognised safe levels. Rainwater itself may contain radioactive materiel (Chernobyl) and acid from various combustion processes. There are frequent reports of the industrial contamination of waterways. This may be due to genuine accident, carelessness or deliberate action. Massive pollution is obvious either by seeing the pollutant itself or by observing the large number of dead fish and other aquatic animals. However I suspect that minimal pollution if commonplace and passes undetected. At present we have to rely upon the Environment Protection Agency to protect our watercourses and to detect, deter and financially penalise the polluters.

Although the technologies exist that can cope with today's polluted waste, I suspect that cost delays their implementation. We still rely upon the use of chlorine, a toxic chemical, to sterilise our water supply. A recent report has suggested that chlorinated drinking water could be linked to the damage of babies prior to birth. Now the British Government would like to introduce fluoride into our drinking water. Fluorine is far more toxic than its sister halogen chlorine, and is one of the most toxic chemicals known. The reason stated is that it could reduce dental decay, but this ignores the safer option of reducing sugar consumption and improving diets through better health education. It has been claimed that both the dental and medical professions have received financial inducements to promote fluoridation of drinking water. How else is it possible for these two professions to ignore some of the evidence presented later in this chapter, and to condone mass compulsory medication at a time when other countries are abandoning their fluoride experiments that have failed to deliver the anticipated dental benefits to offset their many disadvantages? Some countries with the highest use of fluoride also have the most dental cavities.

Fluorine is, as stated above, a very hazardous chemical and the particular compound that they propose to use is an industrial waste product and not the naturally occurring compound. This waste compound contains other very toxic chemicals and all of these chemicals are too toxic to be buried nor dumped at sea. Any use in the fluoridation process of water would spare the manufacturers the highly expensive cost of safe disposal by any other means. All but the very minimal amount added to water could have very serious consequences. Even the recommended concentration has been reported to kill fish in a household aquarium. Accidents can happen as occurred with the aluminium spillage in Cornwall. Following the terrorist attack of September 11th 2001 all potential targets should have had a risk assessment undertaken. Fluoride contamination at a treatment plant would be simple to achieve and catastrophic in its effects, killing possibly thousands of people and animals.

A recent government initiated enquiry intended to reassure the public has been severely criticised for both its terms of reference and the very selective evidence studied. Despite the shortcomings of the enquiry, and its recommendation that further research is needed, government officials are writing to concerned electors claiming that the enquiry had vindicated the proposed fluoridation of our drinking water. Increasing evidence suggests that not only does fluoridation fail to reduce dental cavities, but it also affects bone leading to an increase in fractures of the hip. It has also been implicated in the causation of some cancers. Normal practice in medicine strictly controls the dosage of all medication, especially those medicines that have potentially toxic side effects. Fluoride consumption cannot be controlled because of the wide variation in the consumption of water and fluoride toothpaste. Fluoride can also be absorbed from food cooked in water or even absorbed through the skin when taking a bath. Tea contains fluoride and therefore the consumption of this beverage can also affect the total consumption of this toxic chemical. How can any government, elected to protect the electorate, place their interests second only to the financial health of industry? How too can the medical and dental professions who are dedicated to control the dosage of the drugs that they use even consider supporting mass medication where there is no way to control the amount of fluoride absorbed into the body? Further information is available from either the web site or the newsletters of the National Pure Water Association. In America companies that produce toothpaste, identical to that on sale in the UK, are compelled to add health warnings to the containers. There is general advice about the importance of not swallowing toothpaste. Children under 6 years of age should not use the toothpaste unless directed to do so by a dentist or a doctor. Swallowing of more than a minimal amount should be treated as a medical emergency. No such warnings are required in the UK. Why are we so different?

Even if fluoridation is abandoned, and newer technologies employed, there still remains a potential problem that affects the quality of drinking water. A new organisation, the Centre for Implosion Research, has been formed by two scientists to study the phenomenon of water implosion and has led to a rethink on even the fundamental nature and importance of water. Based upon the original work of the Austrian scientist Viktor Schauberger (1885 – 1958), their work has thrown renewed light upon the character of water. There are several books devoted to the work of this Austrian, but the shortest is "The Schauberger Keys" by Alick Bartholomew. Schauberger claimed that there is a natural cycle to rejuvenate water. Rainwater should slowly percolate through the ground before emerging in underground reservoirs or into rivers. It appears that interruption of this cycle leaves water 'dead' or inert. Oddly enough the UK Government has just issued new planning guidelines (entitled SUDS!) because of concerns over the restricted percolation of rainwater through the ground. We have all seen that water draining from a basin or bath has a natural flow in a spiral, known technically as by implosion. The process of implosion not only reduces friction between water and its containers, but also imparts new life to the water itself. Viktor Schauberger argued that reduced percolation, repeated recycling and being forced through straight pipes further denatures the water. His most sensational claim was that healthy water has the capacity to form a memory of chemicals that it comes into contact with. Professor Jacques Benvenista, Dr Wolfgang Ludwig and David Schweitzer have all claimed to demonstrate that water can store information and picks up negative as well as positive energetic imprints via vibrational transfer. The water's memory thus enables it to both receive and transmit information.

This ability of water to retain the memory of any chemical that it comes into contact with offers a scientific explanation of why homoeopathy is effective. Some people may find this a difficult concept because they consider water to be a simple chemical compound. However although water's memory is of importance to health and to homoeopathy, it does have a downside. It means that water that has been in contact with a toxic chemical will retain the memory of that chemical even after any water treatment process has removed it. This means that the harmful properties will be retained in water. However it is possible that imploded water may be able to convert inorganic chemicals into less toxic organic colloidal ions. This process to form organic ions is essential for the effective absorption of food. Modern experiments using high magnification microscopes and Kirlian photography claim to have demonstrated that molecular changes have occurred in energised water. Experiments with plants exposed to energised water found that there was a 50 percent reduction in feed requirements, stronger root growth and a 250 per cent increase in yield.

The Centre for Implosion Research (www. implosionresearch.com) has developed techniques to energise water and to manufacture various products that are capable of re-energizing any water that they come into contact with. People using imploded water report a variety of benefits. Firstly the taste is improved and also scaling in a kettle, previously used to boil ordinary tap water, will be slowly reabsorbed. It could have the same effects upon all household pipes and also our veins and arteries. Bathing is also reported to be more invigorating.

How significant are the theories of Viktor Schauberger? Certainly Nazi Germany and post war America sought to harness his expertise because they both believed that he could help in the manufacture of nuclear weapons. Sadly today he is only indirectly remembered in the concept of SUDS. If water is so vital to our health why have we allowed government apathy and failure to study the work of this Austrian? Surely our health is more important than the development of weapons of mass destruction? I feel certain that if it were believed that these theories could assist in a weapon program there would be no shortage of available government funds.

Chapter 9

Is Food As Good As It Looks?

*"If we give every individual the right amount of nourishment
and exercise, not too little and not too much, we would have
found the safest way to health"*
(Hippocrates)

Given a choice between food, water and air, most people would
choose food as being the most important. Their decision may be
influenced by the fact that for most people eating would be the
most pleasurable occupation. However the changes in our food
over the past 50 years mirror the general deterioration in health.
History books tell us that diseases like scurvy, pellagra, beriberi
and rickets are caused by inadequate nutrition. Images of starvation are frequently seen on television and in the newspapers.
However harrowing these images may be few people would associate poor nutrition with life in today's Western democracies.
Very few people will experience real hunger. A chosen lifestyle, or
one enforced by financial worries, could lead to an inadequate
diet. However our doctors will tell us that as long as we have a
well balanced diet (whatever that means) we should be consuming all the nutrients that we need, and that supplementation with
vitamins and minerals is not only unnecessary but a waste of
money. It is unfortunate that medical education tends to exclude
information on nutrition, and very few doctors could identify
which diseases are caused by a particular mineral or vitamin deficiency. Of the diseases mentioned above, I would hope that a
diagnosis of rickets could be made with some confidence but I
suspect that scurvy would defy identification. In later chapters
there will be an explanation of the correlation between poor
nutrition and disease. Dr Linus Pauling, a double Nobel Prize
Winner, claimed that it was possible to trace every illness, every
disease and every ailment to a mineral deficiency. An American
doctor claimed that after conducting multiple autopsies on both
animals and humans, that nutritional deficiency was responsible

for all cases of death due to natural causes. I have found that in chronic illness there is always a deficiency of one or more minerals, vitamins or essential fatty acids.

The shops and supermarkets are full of appetising looking food. Fruit for instance may be waxed to increase its eye appeal, and consequently sealing in the toxic herbicides and pesticides used during farming. Many shoppers show signs of obesity rather than malnutrition. It may come as a shock to hear that in general people received a more nutritious diet during the rationing that occurred during World War 2. So if food is so important, and there appears to be abundance available, how can we explain the continual rise in all forms of illness? There has been no attempt to link inadequate nutrition (not to be confused with having insufficient to eat) with this rise in ill health.

Veterinary Surgeons regularly take blood samples from farm animals to ensure that they have sufficient minerals and vitamins. Farmers know that poorly nourished animals may not conceive and successfully deliver their young. That is bad for their farm business. If the same farmer is told that he too is nutritionally deficient he will express surprise, and wonder why his own doctor didn't perform the same blood estimations. Doctors do not ask for these blood tests, and if they do so the hospital laboratories will tell them that they cannot be done. Is it because human health is worth less than the welfare of our farm animals? It is possible that a few charges of professional misconduct resulting from the failure to perform these blood tests could alter the practice of medicine? Perhaps someone with a vested interest in maintaining ill health doesn't like the idea of linking disease to inadequate nutrition? It is worth noting that different races with their different cultures and diets suffer from different diseases. In addition if people move to a different country and then adopt the local diets, they then tend to develop those illnesses that are associated with that new society. Asian women rarely develop such conditions as premenstrual tension in Asia, but they will do so if they move to America and adopt the American lifestyle. Studies in parts of China where there is a chronic deficiency of selenium have noted increased rates of cancer. Adding selenium to the local Chinese diet can reverse this trend. These and other well-documented examples should have alerted western medicine to the crucial role of nutrition in both the prevention and treatment of disease. It should be obvious that good nutrition is the most important factor in maintaining health, and also in reversing the effects of ill health. Therefore the food industry as a whole must bear some of the responsibility for the general decline in health. In the UK the Food Standards Agency seems to have involved itself in almost everything except the most important issue of all, notably the nutritional content of our food.

For thousands of years farmers have known about the importance of crop rotation, and allowing the ground to recover by lying fallow for a year. Of equal importance was to allow animals onto the ground to organically fertilise the earth with their excreta. It was also recognised that flooding of rivers left rich nutrients on the earth. This was why ancient Egypt was so important to invading armies because of the richness of its soil due to the tendency of the river Nile to flood. The sea in the region of the Nile delta used to contain an abundance of fish and other marine life due to the abundant nutritional richness of the waters of the Nile that swept into the sea. In Egypt today the situation has changed because the building of a dam has controlled the flooding. There is now the need to artificially fertilise the land and the inevitable pollution in the outflow of the Nile has led to a depletion of marine life in the region of its delta. Studies in various parts of the world have found that of the various tribes that live to a great age many have rich sources of natural minerals. Their domestic animals are equally healthy and their crops produce the essential vitamins and minerals. In 1936 the American Senate first warned that the soil was becoming depleted of essential vitamins and minerals. Rather than heeding this warning the world embarked upon the production of artificial fertilisers, and more recently artificial herbicides and pesticides. However the concept that man can create artificial products that are as good as, or even better than nature's own, is basically flawed. Industry now believes that it can outperform nature with the GM technology. Plants and animals were designed to utilise natural organic products. Artificial substances may work, or they may be stored and remain unused in the body until sufficient amounts have accumulated to then become toxic and cause harm. In some circumstances, especially in the case of medicines, toxic effects can occur sooner rather than later. In nature it may take hundreds or even thousands of years to evolve and to adapt to environmental change. The ethos of modern chemical manufacturing is to expect such adaptation to occur in a very short period of time (or not to even consider it). Thus man has only himself to blame for so altering his environment that ill health is a natural consequence of his folly. Money and power have assumed an importance and dominance over the needs of man and his environment. Successive governments have stood idly by and allowed the people to be exploited and their health compromised.

Farmers today are often paid by weight for their crops rather than for quality. This has encouraged the use of nitrates and phosphates to boost the yields. We rely upon American grain, not European, which contains these two and other artificial chemicals that are not without their own unwanted adverse side effects. These artificial chemical products are then passed on to the consumer either in the food itself or via water when there is a run off from the fields into the watercourses. These chemicals include artificial herbicides and pesticides that are used to maximise the crop and prevent its reduction by weeds or pests. Recent press reports on pesticides have included: "Pesticide traces in half shop produce", and "Banned pesticides found in fruit and vegetables". Crops can also pose a threat to health because the soil on which they are grown is deficient in many of the essential minerals and vitamins, a fact known to the American Government for nearly seventy years. The British Government has also published data showing the mineral deficiencies of many of the crops grown in the United Kingdom.

The latest technology to be inflicted upon us is the use of genetically modified seed. There have been all sorts of claims made in favour of this technology, including the claim that it is the only way to feed the entire world. This had been disputed by several organisations including the World Health Organisation that states that we already produce double the amount of food needed. In practice this GM technology has created an even

57

greater monopoly by the major seed suppliers. Farmers who use GM seed cannot save some of their harvest as seed for the following year's crops, but are reliant upon the manufacturer for each and every year's supplies of seed. Some western governments have supported this GM project. The bonding between government and industry has been encouraged by the interchanges of personnel between the two. It is not viewed as unacceptable behaviour or as constituting any conflict of interest. In England, despite public opposition, the Labour Government has encouraged genetic farming experiments, and as usual follows America's lead in defying the wishes of its own population and those of the European Union. Neighbouring crops have been contaminated, and organic farmers may no longer be able to make claims to producing organic produce. The consumer may lose the freedom of choice because some of the GM crop may in fact contaminate the produce that is bought labelled as free from all GM ingredients. This is a further example of how governments fail to adequately protect their public, but rather supports the interests of the major industrial corporations. In far too many aspects of today's life, the interests of money and power take precedence over the interest of the public who elect governments. It is perhaps not surprising that so much money is spent to ensure the election of an individual or political party. It is, sadly becoming increasingly necessary to seek the real reason behind any major government initiative.

There are frequent press reports about GM technology. There have been reported comments by a former Environment Minister, Michael Meacher expressing his real concerns. There have been complaints that a prominent unelected minister, with substantial financial interests in GM technology, has been allowed to sit in on cabinet discussions on implementing GM food production. Included here is a selection of recent articles. "GM seed blunder deepens public doubts". "Stop the GM zombies" referring to a Watchdog report on pigs and cows being bred to feel no stress. "Mutant pollen is spread by GM crop that wouldn't die". "The secret plan to combine GM seeds with normal crops". "Alarm over the GM mutant weed" "GM blunder contaminates Britain with mutant crops". "Just how far has GM crop pollution spread?"

Earlier in this chapter, I claimed that in many ways people were better nourished during the days of rationing that occurred during World War 2. There appear to be four main reasons for this. Firstly, the food was generally produced locally and, secondly, it was generally consumed whilst fresh. Thirdly, agriculture hadn't at that time become a major industry with large farms, increased mechanisation and reliance upon artificial chemicals. Lastly, food was only eaten when in season.

In rural parts of those countries around the Mediterranean Sea, whose lifestyle and health many of us envy, these four features still persist. However today's sophisticated consumers now wants access to their preferred foods all year round. This in turn leads to greater choice of inferior quality produce. This now means that food is brought from all over the world to end up in our shops and supermarkets. There is no UK control of the food's development and uninvited contaminants may also be imported. In some previously rural economies, the demand for this greater all year round production, geared to the export of produce, has caused a fall off in natural nutrition and consequently a greater reliance upon selective artificial fertilisers. The food must eventually end up in our food stores in an attractive condition. This means that some fruit must be picked unripe and artificially ripened when reaching the eventual destination. Even then food may be stored for up to two years before going on sale. In one experiment oranges were tracked on their journey from Spain to the shelves of UK stores. Vitamin C levels were measured at various stages in the journey from the orange groves and it was found that at the point of sale there was virtually no vitamin C left in the oranges. Remember that lack of vitamin C causes scurvy, and it is no use eating lots of oranges and expecting to remain free of colds throughout the winter. If you don't trust elaborate experiments and trials then I suggest that the next time you travel to Spain, France or Italy just sample the local fruit that is in season and see if there is any difference in taste.

So it is as well to remember that the next time you admire the fresh fruit and vegetables in your local supermarket, what you see is certainly not fresh. Furthermore it is no use relying upon these products to provide you with your daily requirements of vitamins and minerals, so if you wish to remain healthy and achieve longevity you will need to take supplements. I advise everyone to ignore advice that minerals and vitamins are either worthless or dangerous until doctors are forced to estimate a patient's nutritional status. The old adage of "an apple a day keeps the doctor away" no longer applies. In general we rely upon plants to manufacture the vitamins that are so essential to our good health. The plants themselves cannot manufacture these vitamins unless all the minerals are present in the soil that surrounds their roots. Experiments using organic mineral supplementation, especially when fulvic acid is added, show a marked difference between those plants that are fed in this manner and those that are not. Fulvic acid is a natural substance found around plant roots that aids in breaking down minerals so that they are easily absorbed into the plant. Thereafter fulvic acid appears to assist in the transport of nutrients into the cells and then aids the elimination of waste.

Please don't allow the government, the food industry and your doctors to deceive you into believing that what you see buy and consume is both safe and contains all your nutritional requirements.

Chapter 10

Is The Meat And Fish We Buy
Safe To Eat?

There are two main reasons why we should pay more attention to the practice of livestock farming. Firstly, and most obviously, we need to know exactly what we are eating and especially, what we should avoid. Secondly, we ought to apply the lessons learnt during the recent farming disasters to help in the treatment and prevention of human disease.

We have already seen that commercial considerations dictate the methods of food production. The intention is to produce a wide range of appealing products at a competitive price, but to leave a reasonable profit margin. Like any other commercial product, food is marketed by advertising. Often medical and health claims are utilised to promote a food product. On some occasions doctors themselves are targeted to encourage them to advise patients on the various merits of a particular food. Regrettably differing research and advertising claims can leave the consumer confused and often misinformed. Every attempt is made to influence the buying habits of the consumer, in what to buy and where to purchase it. "An apple a day keeps the doctor away", "go to work on an egg" and "drink a pint of milk a day" are all examples of early attempts to influence the consumer. Eventually the promotions became more sophisticated as witnessed by the debates on cholesterol and saturated versus unsaturated fatty acids. This was incorporated into a campaign to persuade us to use margarine in preference to butter.

Once the demand for a product has been established by advertising and promotion, production has to be increased by commercially viable means. This has led to a remarkable change in farming methods and the transformation of the traditional rural economy by a process similar to that of the industrial revolution. Big farms are now considered more desirable, and money has been poured into agriculture to create large commercial farms.

Highly sophisticated and mechanised food production factories have replaced the small and labour intensive farms. The former rural way of life has been largely destroyed in order to achieve a more plentiful supply of food at a more competitive price. However there is evidence that, as mentioned in the previous chapter, quality has been sacrificed in order to achieve greater quantities of food.

Thus the intensive farming of livestock was created. This has meant that animals have been crowded into small confined pens or stalls. As a consequence there have been continual clashes with the various animal rights organisations. Crowding together of animals has increased the risks of infection spreading rapidly through the stock. Hence the routine, and indiscriminate, administration of antibiotics. At a time when indiscriminate use of antibiotics in human medicine is being discouraged, consumption of livestock products exposes people to a variety of antibiotics and possibly even drug resistant bacteria. Salmonella infection from eggs, and food poisoning associated with the consumption of chickens has been well documented. There have also been several well-publicised epidemics of E.Coli infection associated with the consumption of beef. Other causes of food poisoning include Lysteria and Campylobacter. Pigs are scavengers and therefore consumption of pork exposes people to all sorts of infections and toxic substances. Many animal infections are from organisms other than bacteria and therefore the use of antibiotics is worthless.

People are now exposed to antibiotics, drug resistant organisms, non-bacterial infections and other chemicals including hormones and cortisones that are used to promote animal growth. Not surprisingly, food poisoning continues to increase, although it is not always reported. In February 2003 the Food Standards Agency reported that there were 5 million people affected in 2000, 5.5 million in 2001 and 6 million in 2002. This equates to one in ten people being subject to food poisoning every year. In my experience many affected people do not consult their doctor, who in turn may feel that the illness is not linked to food poisoning. One reason that the Food Agency was formed was to achieve a reduction in the numbers of people suffering from food poisoning. This epidemic is estimated to cost this Country £750 million per year. Furthermore, evidence from Danish research suggests the death rate due to food poisoning is far higher than previously thought. Poor techniques at slaughterhouses, poor personal hygiene, improperly cooked meat and mixing cooked and raw products together, also carry increased risks of food poisoning. In today's world, we should expect a reduction in the number of cases of food poisoning, or are we all guilty of cutting corners in the belief that modern medical treatment will cure any resulting problem? In a later chapter the unsuspected epidemic of parasites is documented, and animals are a potent source of parasites. The BSE epidemic demonstrated how easily infection can spread amongst animals, and how poor slaughterhouse techniques can lead to human infection producing a ticking time bomb with no one as yet sure how many people will eventually succumb to the associated human illnesses. Some days we are told that thousands, or even millions of people are likely to be affected, on other days we are reassured that the threat to human health has been grossly overestimated.

Intensive farming requires a variety of animal foodstuffs. Usually animals are fed with a variety of substances that are generally not found in their natural diet. Thus animals, like human beings, are fed substances that are alien to their natural diet developed over many hundreds of years, and they are expected to adapt to this change without any undesirable consequences. Animal feed constitutes a major cost for intensive farmers, because animals are expected to achieve a given weight before they can go to market to be slaughtered. Animals kept in confined spaces expend fewer calories on energy, leaving the remainder to achieve weight gain. Administration of hormones, including oestrogens, corticosteroids and growth hormones are added to the feed to boost the rate of weight gain. Although medicine is beginning to appreciate the possible dangers of such chemicals as yet they haven't been banned in the rearing of animals. Once again it is worth stressing that these are synthetic chemicals that are not normally found in the bodies of both animals and humans. Some counties have banned certain chemicals that are made in America, that are used to increase milk yield in cows, because of fears that they may cause cancer. However this has led to trade disputes with the American Government that has championed the use of such products. There are very strong links between the American Administration and these companies. We are what we eat and therefore the quality of our food is vital. If we eat such affected produce we also consume the various chemicals that have been fed to the animals during their lifetime.

There have been various investigative television programmes that have shown how animals that have been condemned as unfit for human consumption, nevertheless end up in the shops and on sale to the public. Is it any wonder that the number of cases of food poisoning continues to rise when financial interests are yet again rated higher than human health? Perhaps if we had adopted a more moral view of animal welfare we could have been repaid by an improvement in human health. Nature has a habit of fighting back whenever we feel that we can do things better.

There are several diseases that can have a profound effect upon the farming community. Some like Foot and Mouth, BSE and Swine Fever in pigs reach the national headlines. Nobody can be unaffected by the sight of burning carcasses of the slaughtered animals. For many small farmers it can spell financial ruin. There are similar diseases that can decimate flocks of chickens and turkeys.

Perhaps it would be worthwhile making a closer look at the issues surrounding BSE and Foot and Mouth disease. The scandal of BSE refuses to go away. Slaughterhouse conditions have already been mentioned. Although the infective agent is not fully understood, we were wrongly reassured that there was no danger to public health. There is also a large question mark over various foodstuffs including the use of infected material from other diseased animals. Foodstuffs banned for use in this country were subsequently sold abroad, leading to the infection of Continental herds. There is a question mark over the actions of the various authorities. There is now the suggestion that animals could, or should be vaccinated against BSE. Vaccines do not always contain exactly the identical organism that is found in a disease, and it is not yet known just how effective they are, and anyway do we need to consume yet another unwanted chemical? Human studies have shown that the complications caused by vaccines can then be passed from mother to unborn infant; therefore it is possible to assume the possible passage from cow to calf and thence once again to humans. Cattle are herbivores, used to roaming the fields, and so is it any wonder that confining them to pens and feeding them a variety of animal by-products and chemicals causes problems like BSE? Certain feeds derived from diseased sheep were banned from use in cattle, but found their way into chicken and fish farms.

Foot and Mouth disease is another disease that can spread rapidly from farm to farm. The infective agent is a virus, and again the possibility of using vaccines has been raised. However, in a later chapter, the use of homoeopathic anti-viral agents is mentioned. We know that homoeopathic remedies are very effective in animals, and carry no threat if the animal is cured and subsequently passed for human consumption. As in BSE the methods of disposal were incineration and burial. In both these diseases there is the possibility of airborne toxins associated with incineration, and pollution by seepage in the case of burial. In the region of London's old Covent Garden excavation below basement level is discouraged because it is a former burial site for victims of the plague. In addition it has been argued that these epidemics, and their mismanagement, were engineered to reduce a perceived excess of cattle and to reduce the numbers of small farmers in order to create larger and more commercial farms. Who knows the real truth?

Another condemnation of modern farming techniques comes from research in India. There, one farmer paid special attention to the welfare of his cattle following his prior selection of healthy stock. Attention was paid to their stalls including fresh bedding. Proper feedstuffs were used. These healthy cattle, with an effective immune system, were then exposed to cattle infected with Foot and Mouth disease. Apart from a few blisters there were no adverse effects and these healthy cattle survived. Therein lies the moral and perhaps the reasons why the general health of both livestock and humans has deteriorated: falling levels of immunity. In yet another example a Scandinavian Government, responding to the pressure from animal welfare groups, introduced animal welfare legislation. Legal minimal standards of accommodation were introduced along with food guidelines and a restriction upon the use of antibiotics and various chemical hormones products. There were initially protests from the farming lobby at the perceived additional financial costs of these proposals. Subsequently, it proved that there were increasing and not decreasing profits and that, furthermore, the consumer benefited because of the improved quality of the farm produce. In both arable and livestock farming there are many unanswered questions regarding the actions of governments, intensive farmers and the various major corporations that supply the farming industry.

In the study of food we mustn't forget the harvest of the sea. Fish has always been considered to be a safe and healthy food. The only major concern has been the shortage of fish as a result of over fishing. However there is growing concern about the safety of fish. There have been several examples were pollution of rivers and lakes has led to anatomical abnormalities of fish and other marine animals. These are mainly relating to the sex of the fish, male fish becoming more feminine in appearance. In addition to the congenital abnormalities there is the possibility that lack of fertility could threaten future fish production. These abnormalities have been associated with accidental spillage, or even deliberate pollution with various chemicals related to the female hormone, oestrogen. There is also evidence that polar bears are suffering similar abnormalities. Unfortunately the oceans of the world have been used for dumping unwanted substances ranging from untreated sewage to industrial and radioactive waste. This dumping has until recently attracted little opposition from governments. Due to the various sea currents certain areas seem to attract greater concentrations of these pollutants. The North Sea is one such area that appears to have greater concentrations of various pollutants. This was highlighted by French research that tracked the progress of radioactive discharge from the reprocessing plant at Cap de la Hague on the Cherbourg peninsular. They found that the radioactive discharge passed up the west coast of England, then north of Scotland and eventually ending up in the North Sea. This radioactive migration was probably joined by any discharge from

Sellafield. Therefore any fish in the North Sea swim in a cocktail of radioactive, industrial and human waste.

The French researchers also followed the progress of radioactivity through the fish food chain and found that some species concentrated more of the radioactive waste than others. It was been known for some time that Tuna had been polluted with abnormal levels of mercury. In February 2003 pregnant mothers were officially warned to limit their consumption of tinned tuna because the mercury it contained posed a risk to their unborn children. Ironically, another government department tried to reassure parents that the mercury levels in many vaccines posed no threat to their children. There is clear evidence that the total amount of mercury injected directly into children as part of the vaccination programme exceeds the safety levels for this metal. Despite the claims regarding its safety, some manufacturers have been encouraged to cease using this toxic metal as a preservative for their vaccines. In France the transport of mercury needs a police escort!! Other fish products including the popular liver oils have been implicated as being potentially contaminated with various pollutants, including dioxins.

In an effort to make up for possible shortage of fish from the seas, a new industry of fish farming has sprung up. Fish from these farms had a definite consumer appeal. However the fish farmers have failed to learn from the mistakes of intensive animal farmers. In recent months there has been increasing evidence that fish from these farms are becoming diseased. Swimming in confined spaces along with their own excreta and artificial feed (even similar to the feed associated with BSE in cattle) it is no wonder that such fish are prone to diseases. Recent press reports have single out farmed salmon as being affected by these conditions. These farmed salmon appear to have 20 percent more fat than their wild cousins. There is also evidence that the diseases that affect these farmed fish are now spreading to infect the wild fish swimming in the neighbouring waters.

There is definite concern about the quality and safety of much of the produce for human consumption. Hazards to health don't cease when leaving the farms, because there are further potential health risks during the journey before the produce reaches your home. This journey will be the subject of the next chapter. There is a clear comparison between the illnesses endured by animals and fish reared under intensive farming techniques and human health when we not only eat the compromised products but also to share the same polluted environment.

Chapter 11

Food And Its Travels

Food has to make a hazardous journey from its source of production until it ends up on the plate and ready to be eaten. In the two previous chapters it was noted that on many occasions the quality of food was suspect even before it left its point of origin. This chapter deals with its processing and journey to the retail outlet and its time spent on the shelf prior to purchase. There is legislation designed to protect the consumer. However, there is often insufficient inspection to ensure that the legislation is complied with. In addition there are gaps in the law, and quite often there are delays in bringing forward new regulations or advice on known risks. In the last chapter there was the example of toxic levels of mercury in tuna. This fact was known for some considerable time before it was drawn to the public's attention and pregnant women advised to restrict their consumption of this fish. Another example has been the failure to warn the public about the contamination of various fish oil products.

In the last chapter it was mentioned that there have been several examples of meat products, condemned as unfit for human consumption that had nevertheless reached both shops and restaurants enabling dishonest traders to make substantial profits. Even meat that has been passed as fit for human consumption can have its safety compromised by poor hygiene during its processing. Most local Councils are having budget shortfalls and therefore tend to restrict the numbers of both environmental and trading standards officers. Quite often these local government officials are overwhelmed with work, especially if they work in a tourist area that has large numbers of hotels and restaurants. Similarly there are increased pressures associated with the presence of large numbers of meat processing plants. It is also very difficult to control the quality, type and composition of products like sausages pies and burgers. In the case of these processed meat products, there is the added need to ensure that the labelling is both accurate and not misleading.

Food is also treated to increase its visual appeal, to enhance its flavour and often to extend its shelf life. A plethora of E number additives has been introduced during recent years. These have led to an increase in the numbers of people becoming sensitive to these chemicals. Time spent watching the habits of shoppers will demonstrate how many people now closely examine the list of ingredients because of their own known sensitivities. One example is the food enhancer known as mono sodium glutamate (MSG), which is commonly used in Chinese cooking and also in very many processed foods. With increasing sensitivity to MSG, most Chinese restaurants, when asked, will now cook without using this chemical. However this is not always possible because some food items are marinated in MSG before they are cooked. Many people suffer from indigestion after eating white bread that has chemicals added to maintain its freshness for several days. These same people may remain symptom free when eating Continental white bread that only lasts for 5 hours before losing its freshness. Few people will be unaware that an unfortunate number of people are very sensitive to peanuts, and that they can suffer a life threatening allergic reaction if they eat this particular nut. It is now quite common to see warning notices that an item either contains peanuts or that there could be some contamination by this particular nut during processing or cooking. If there is any doubt, customers are advised to seek additional information from a waiter or shop worker. Unfortunately sometimes reassuring advice is given in error because the advice does not come from a chef or similar person in authority.

We read that scientists are working upon the production of a GM peanut that can avoid allergic or hypersensitive reactions. This then begs several questions. Will all the existing peanut plants be taken out of production and replaced by the new GM variety? Will there be separate areas for the cultivation of the GM plants, and who will guarantee that the two varieties don't become mixed together? If this technology does materialise then the cost of peanuts is certain to rise. The more fundamental mistake is that due a failure to understand the underlying causes of allergy, the patient is likely to develop new allergies once the original peanut sensitivity has been removed. It is therefore theoretically possible to become sensitive to the GM peanut!

With our changed lifestyles there has been an increase in the number of so-called fast food restaurants and also the sale of convenience foods. It is debatable whether this industry sprang up in response to changing lifestyles, or caused the changes to take place. These ready to cook meals can be used in the home, without the need for preparation, and can be ready for consumption in a very short time. Some restaurant chains that have a standardised menu have chilled/frozen meals that can be cooked in the microwave in a very short space of time. This can even include such dishes as pre-prepared omelettes. The effect of microwave cooking is dealt with elsewhere. If you are doubt about how your meal is cooked, always ask. However don't been too reassured by the expression 'home cooked' because this often means that the packet or tin has been opened in the kitchen. The real clue as to what happens in the kitchen is to look for the 'staff required' adverts, and if they are seeking a microwave technician rather than a chef then you can be sure that your meal was prepared and cooked many miles away and possibly even days beforehand. Irradiation of uncooked food to increase its shelf life is another hidden hazard.

Manufacturers of processed foods have to ensure that their products are both appetising to look at, tasty to eat and inexpensive to manufacture. This has led to the regular use of both sugar and salt that in turn has resulted in some people consuming these two chemicals in excess. The dangers of the two substances have been well documented. The medical profession and various nutritional bodies have been drawing attention to these dangers. However habits and tastes have been established and it will take a concerted effort by governments and the various regulatory bodies to reverse the trend. At last the present Government has acknowledged the links between these foods, obesity and an increase in many other diseases with their associated reduction in life expectancy. Lists of ingredients don't seem to excite public awareness unless there is a crisis like BSE and the possibility of products like beef burgers posing a health hazard.

Another ingredient that poses a health problem is animal fat and its excessive use in processed foods. There is too much reliance upon these fats that may contain some of the toxins or infectious agents that were present in the animals prior to slaughter. This in turn adds to the health threats posed by the use of excess salt and sugar. So far no government seems anxious to control and regulate these foods, and chooses or prefers to ignore the consequences to public health and national wealth. Perhaps the balance has swung too far in favour of vested interests and the perceived financial need to curtail longevity.

There is however another section of the food industry that caters for those people who wish to lose weight or to remain thin. Having established a taste for sweet foods and realising that sugar, which is usually of the more harmful refined type, contributes to weight gain, there has been a search for alternatives that would retain the sweet taste. Therefore a variety of sweeteners has been manufactured and are widely used in low calorie foods and drinks. These include such chemicals as aspartame, which has long been recognised as being potentially toxic and carcinogenic. A large American company manufactures this chemical and no action has been taken by that country to limit its production. The European Commission has sought to impose restrictions upon the use of these sweeteners. Once again the American Government is trying to compel the European Community to lift this ban. It is amazing that the American people themselves fail to force their own Government to ban this and similar chemicals. It is surprising that a complacent American public realises and accepts the apparent corruption in politics and big business, and does nothing to correct it. Stevia, a natural sweetener that is available in America is ironically banned in the UK. Many diet drinks are also sparkling, and many youngsters can drink up to 20 cans/bottles of these products in a single day. The chemicals that create these bubbles can have a destabilising effect upon the bodies' mineral balances. One consequence of this is the occurrence of osteoporosis in both sexes from a very early age. Although this increase in osteoporosis is causing alarm and increasing financial pressure upon the health services, there is little or no effort made to discourage the consumption of these beverages. In some women this osteoporosis and the lack of adequate physical exercise suggests that their lives will be marred by illness from an early age, and even possibly premature death. Hospitals should lead by example and refuse to allow the sale of these products within their buildings. It is astounding that the Labour Government is encouraging hospitals to make available convenience food and drinks, including crisps and sparkling liquids, readily available for the consumption of patients within the wards.

Correct and accurate labelling of food products is essential, and various pieces of legislation have been passed in an attempt to protect the public. Sell by dates are required, but again need to be enforced. In this respect the customer should now be its own inspector. If there is a lack of satisfaction then the local Trading Standards Officer should be informed. The authorities are becoming increasingly vigilant in stopping misleading labels. "Juice firms face squeeze on labels", relates to a requirement not to claim pure fruit when there is a dilution of concentrated fruit with water. The containers should contain the exact article as stated on the label. If the product is expensive as in the case of pure olive oil, there is always the temptation to dilute or substitute as occurred in Spain several years ago. Overheating a cooking oil can lead to the formation of carcinogenic chemicals. In recent months Germany banned the sale of a particular English manufactured crisp bread because of concerns that the oil used in the manufacture could have been overheated and therefore harmful. It is believed that the crisp bread company concerned has altered its manufacturing process.

Direct and indirect advertising of products also causes concern. There has, for some time been the concern that the cinema and television glorifies the consumption of alcohol and the smoking of tobacco products. Now the authorities are beginning to turn their attention to the foods. "Bob the fat builder" was the title of an article criticising the BBC for using popular TV characters to help the sale of junk food. However in reality it is very difficult to police the food processing and sales industries. There should be control over the advertising of fats, salts and sugar and those foods that are considered detrimental to health. There should be effective monitoring to ensure that there is no subtle advertising of these products by including their prominent use during programs. The food industry has diversified and expanded so rapidly that it has proved impossible to police every single type or specific food. There are also many different legal requirements and too many agencies authorised to enforce them. Perhaps the education authorities made the single most damaging decision when the first efforts were made to reduce their budgets. Many schools stopped providing lunches leading to the culture of cold, pre-packed junk food meals. Furthermore, education authorities by and large decided that health education was not a core subject. The Labour Government has introduced a healthy eating programme, but failed to put it actually into practice with lessons, instructions and books. In consequence a whole new generation has grown up without any real knowledge of health nutrition and cooking. These are the parents of today who have no knowledge to pass onto their own children. These families now have to rely upon television and advertisements for their information, and then consequently adopt the lifestyles as portrayed by their role models. The Foods Standard Agency says there is no need for supplements if you eat a 'balanced diet'. Their definition of a balanced diet is a little of everything built around 'starchy foods', plus 5 lots of fruit and vegetables per day. The French advise 10 portions of vegetables per day. The tragedy is that many English children don't recognise all fruit and vegetables, let alone eat them. The charity CANCERactive is working with Michelle Roe and Sheila Gaukroger, who have already run three pilot tests in the North East of England. These two ladies aim to provide lessons, books and other educational tools to supplement the present school curriculum. I am anxious to see if this scheme can be introduced into my local schools.

No concern for an individual's own health can exclude knowledge of the food chain from source to dinner table. How is it produced, is it contaminated, does it contain all the minerals and vitamins that are needed, how fresh is it, is it part of a balanced diet and finally once bought has it been properly stored and cooked in a manner that hasn't destroyed its vitality?

There are powerful arguments against governments exerting too much control over our daily lives. However they have a responsibility to ensure the maintenance of our health. They have sufficient legislation in place, but they must ensure that it is enforced. The present emphasis on the education system should have included a requirement that everyone should be capable of making an informed choice about their own, and their family's health. So far successive governments have failed their people.

Chapter 12

Do Charities Really Care?

Charities have been a feature of our society for a very long time. Some, like the RSPCA and the NSPC, are recognised and respected both nationally and internationally. Their aims and ethics are both patently obvious and laudable. Like other charities they are regulated by the Charity Commissioners and have to produce authenticated accounts. The Charity Commission has to ensure that they are properly administered, and the inspection of a charity's affairs can be very thorough and time consuming. The Commission isn't required to form an opinion about the aims and objectives of an individual charity, but it has to ensure that the monies raised are properly accounted for. However there appears to no control on how much of the income is spent on the stated good works. I was once told by a volunteer for a large national charity that she would still be happy if only 1 per cent of the money raised eventually reached the people in need of that charity's help.

The close association between medicine and a number of charities has existed for very many years. However the numbers of charities allied to medicine has mushroomed in the past few decades, and has mirrored the increased incidence in chronic ill health and the increased number of diagnostic categories that have been a feature of modern medical practice. These new categories of disease often result from minute changes in the symptoms or diagnostic tests. These changes could be as a result of a normal evolutionary process, or even the result of medical intervention itself, which can cause an alteration in symptoms that in turn, can lead to a new diagnosis. The publication in a medical journal of these new symptoms, and consequently a new diagnosis can lead to wider recognition for the author, and even the possibility that the author's own name could be used to describe this 'new medical condition'.

Prior to the introduction of the present state run health care systems, charities existed to enable poorer patients to obtain medical care. Charity funding in the past has also helped to support the building and running of many hospitals. I can remember seeing the nameplates of donors above individual hospital beds. Other charities helped to fund improved living and working conditions of both resident nurses and doctors. With the advent of the NHS many hospitals and their supporting charities were forced to find new ways in which to channel their funds into the functioning of these institutions. Today most hospitals are associated with a variety of charitable organisations. These charities may help to support specific types of patient, or specific departments of the hospital. Many hospitals now rely upon charities to purchase specific pieces of equipment, or even to fund, or part fund, the salary of a member of staff. The equipment may range from a particular small, but specialised instrument, to a larger machine costing in excess of £1,000,000. Whatever the moral view that medicine should be funded only via the state, it is now a reality that these charities are essential to maintain hospitals' ability to cope with an increasing demand due to increasing levels of ill health that a drug based practice of medicine is not only incapable halting, but also even adding to the size of problem. The change in the attitude of the NHS towards charities since 1948 is remarkable. Then any charity money was frowned upon, and not a little ingenuity was required to spend the charities proceeds. Nowadays executive and non-executive directors of NHS Trusts play an active part in these charities. Scrutiny of these charity funds are included within the hospital's own accounts, and are frequently commented upon by the various audit bodies. However it is difficult to find a charity willing to fund research into the role of nutrition in the cause and prevention of disease. Similarly it is difficult to find research funding into alternative therapies.

Although the financial affairs of charities are scrutinised by various organisations, perhaps it is time that there was additional scrutiny, especially of medical charities. Perhaps it is time to introduce legislation that leads to wider scrutiny to include the aims and objectives, and perhaps the morals of medical charities that compete for our financial contributions.

Charities have now become big business. The majority of High

Streets now rely upon a number of charity shops to fill vacant premises, which helps to convey a sense of prosperity and financial viability, or even the very survival of a shopping centre. These charity shops trade at a distinct advantage because their overheads are much reduced because of savings on commercial rates, many staff are volunteers and the goods are often free or bought at a reduced cost. The profits are then ploughed into the funds of that charity.

Cancer related charities are now some of the biggest and best organised institutions. Within the realm of these medical charities by far the largest amount of money is directed into research for the treatment of cancer. This research into the treatment of cancer is invariably focused on a drug-based approach. If a doctor or therapist makes a claim that they can cure cancer, then they are reprimanded in some manner. However a charity is allowed to ask for money by stating that, "together we can cure cancer." A breast cancer charity can claim "Research cures cancer. Research needs your money." Far from curing breast cancer there appears to an ever-increasing incidence of this particular disease! The relationship between the drug companies and the charities is far too close. Drug companies often sponsor charity fund raising events, whilst in their turn charities help to sponsor drug trials.

Throughout the world the total money raised by these charities and other organisations is devoted to treatment of disease, yet only a miniscule amount of money is spent upon the education necessary to **prevent** cancer. There is no profit for the drug industry, nor glory for charities, in the prevention of cancer, nor indeed for any other chronic disease. Both these organisations expend a considerable amount of time and money to place obstacles in the path of natural therapies (the potential for success using these therapies are described in later chapters).

At a recent charity event, which was sponsored by a drug company, a doctor was pleading for financial contributions. He uses drugs to treat cancer, and his plea for more money was based upon the fact that there had been an increase in the number of patients needing his help. The company sponsoring the event manufactures many of the drugs used by that doctor. Perhaps the doctor should have asked himself why he and many other doctors are faced by an ever-increasing number of cancer patients. It never seems to occur to them that this could represent a failure of their favoured treatment, and that they should seek other ways that might include more effort at preventing disease.

More importantly researchers, who are funded by charities or drug companies, whose results appear to oppose the perceived wisdoms of their paymasters, are often 'rewarded' by having their research grants terminated and in some cases also their employment. Hospital based research is now almost totally funded and directed by the pharmaceutical industry and charities, and inevitably results in the adoption by hospitals of the new therapy, which is invariably more expensive, probably no more effective and most likely to have even more dangerous side effects.

Other charities exist to offer advice, comfort, education and support to patients who suffer from a variety of chronic illnesses. These charities are increasing in number to match not only the mushrooming number of new diagnoses, but also to cope with those diseases such as autism, which were at one time rarely seen but are today quite commonly found. Some of these charities offer money into the research of their specific illness. Once again little or no money is offered into research of preventative measures. However bizarre it may sound some charities may resist any attempt to prevent or cure their particular disease, especially if it is by the use of natural substances, which are therefore free from patent. It appears that the continued existence of the charity, and those people who work for it, are of more importance than the interests of the patients. I have come across several examples of this practice. For example:

- A young male patient suffered a particularly severe form of arthritis. He was no longer able to work, and stayed at home to help look after his young family when his wife had to become the full time breadwinner. Conventional treatments failed, and so he placed an article in the local newspaper asking for help. We saw him, treated his underlying viral infection, and this led to recovery and his ability to return to employ-

79

ment. He was so grateful and full of newfound energy that he threw himself into efforts to help other fellow sufferers. He then became actively involved in the local branch of the appropriate national charity. As a result he organised a local symposium and arranged for a variety of leading experts to attend. The national charity encouraged and helped with the organisation of this meeting. However at the last minute he was prevented from allowing any alternative practitioners to speak. This effectively prevented him from sharing his experiences with other arthritic sufferers.

- Another charity holds an annual essay competition. This is open to both lay and professional entrants. An essay detailing how sufferers could be either cured, or at least helped by the use of natural remedies, was rejected for not being in accordance with the aims of the charity although it was in line with the subject matter chosen for that particular year. The decision to reject the essay was apparently taken by two doctors. This deprived the very many people who rely upon this charity, from being able to judge for themselves if the facts within the rejected essay were relevant to them.

- The number of children suffering from autism is increasing at an alarming rate. One of the charities devoted to this subject also arranges seminars, which are intended to expand the knowledge of this disease. An offer to contribute a lecture on the possible role of vaccination in this disease was rejected because other speakers might cover the subject in their lectures. There was no mention of this topic in the published agenda, neither was there any mention of the effects of mineral and vitamin deficiencies. The deficiencies associated with autism are capable of proof if medicine would contemplate routine estimation of blood samples for specific minerals and vitamins. There is the argument that they are incapable of being measured yet, as previously mentioned Veterinary Surgeons perform assays of these same minerals and vitamins almost routinely on farm animals. Therefore we are forced to conclude that some charities too have a vested interest in maintaining, or even increasing, the number of sufferers.

Other charities actively encourage lectures from a broad spectrum of speakers. Quite often these charities are organised and run by the sufferers themselves who have a vested interest in getting relief from their symptoms. The Hyperactive Children's Support Group is an excellent example of a charity dedicated to the support of its members. They are available to offer advice, help and a shoulder to weep on. When they hold seminars they invite a wide range of speakers, including nutritional researchers, and with both orthodox and alternative practitioners. I am sure that this particular charity would welcome a reduction in the numbers of affected children.

PART 2
The Solutions

*"When diet is wrong medicine is of no use.
When diet is correct medicine is of no need"*

Ancient Ayurvedic proverb

Chapter 13

Lifestyle:
The First Step On The Road To Health

With the knowledge gained from this book and from the other sources of information mentioned within it, it is possible to make an informed decision about your future lifestyle: what you can embrace and what you choose to disregard. Of course different people will come to widely differing conclusions. Sadly, the majority of individuals will only make their choice following a diagnosis of life-threatening ill health. A lifestyle change is only the first, but major, step on the road to achieving and then maintaining good health. Sometimes these lifestyle changes are all that is necessary, but often, additional help is needed. In the following chapters these other barriers to health are explained, and more importantly how they are overcome.

Please remember that a diagnosis is worthless when coming to a conclusion regarding the cause of some acute and all chronic illness. Two medical colleagues have expressed their grave reservations with this statement. They both argue that the early diagnosis of cancer is vital for a patient to have a reasonable chance of survival. Although I have some sympathy with this point of view, their opinion is only fully justified if cancer is not only a distinct and unique entity but also if surgery, radiotherapy and chemotherapy are the only treatments available to doctors. In this book I suggest that cancer is no different from other chronic diseases, and that all these diseases represent the inevitable outcome that results from some other underlying pathology. My theory proposes that a cancer patient that survives surgery, radiotherapy and chemotherapy is likely to suffer from the same unsuspected pathology that was responsible for the formation of the cancer itself. Therefore if the underlying pathology is not treated the patient is unlikely to regain full health and will remain prone to a reoccurrence of the cancer, or even to develop some other chronic illness. This theory has serious implications for most forms of statistical research and also the comparisons between various treatments. The research is only valid if comparisons are made between treatments and outcomes of the underlying pathology and not the perceived diagnoses of modern medicine. There will be further examples in later chapters but two examples are worth making now. If osteoporosis is the result of boron or magnesium deficiency then what is the point of comparing chemical or natural hormone therapy in patients with normal hormone levels? If a cancer has been the result of selenium deficiency caused by an alcohol-excreting parasite, then on completion of conventional treatment the patient will still be selenium deficient and still suffer the effects of an alcohol-excreting parasite

Diagnosis is made following routine medical history, examination and investigations. A recent study of post mortem findings in patients who had died in a hospital intensive care unit discovered that 40 per cent of the original diagnoses were incorrect. This is despite the fact that intensive care units have some of the best equipment and also a high proportion of highly qualified doctors. I remember a similar percentage of incorrect diagnoses found at post mortem when I was a student. Therefore it is safe to assume that a similar, if not greater, proportion of errors occur outside hospitals. Its main function is to provide a name and classification for the disease in question, which is then used to hunt for appropriate drugs, listed in a catalogue of pharmaceutical products. A worldwide vice-president of genetics at Glaxo-SmithKline is quoted as saying that fewer than half of the patients prescribed some of the most expensive drugs actually derived any benefit from them. However there was no shareholder panic because it was suggested that genetic engineering would be the new money generating treatment for disease, and he was speaking as vice-president of genetics. As mentioned elsewhere, arthritis, ME, IBS, stress and the menopause are all examples of worthless diagnoses, and that pharmaceutical products are designed to alleviate symptoms and not to cure or to prevent illness.

Ill health is usually the stimulus that drives the patient, relatives and friends, to discover for themselves more about the illness. They usually receive little or no official help in their search for answers. Is this official negligence, complacency, ignorance or a deliberate conspiracy of silence? This condemns people to prolonged ill health. Governments rigidly support the official health care system despite mounting evidence of its failures. Nothing in medicine is 100 per cent safe, not even the humble aspirin. Despite this, governments and their scientific advisers will continue to maintain that an individual product or a procedure is 100 per cent safe, and that it poses no threat to the public. The more modern the pharmaceutical product, the more likely the possibility of unwanted and possibly dangerous side effects.

If you have come to read this book because you are in good health and that you wish to remain so by preventing the development of disease, then congratulations. Sadly, too many people seek help only when it is almost too late. Everyone, including doctors, espouses the notion that prevention is better than cure, but regrettably too few people choose to practice what they preach. Choosing a healthy lifestyle is a prime example of practicing prevention. Quite often the tools of prevention are the same as the tools of treatment leading to a cure, rather than to the suppression of symptoms. The National Health Service is far too busy in coping with illness to spare time and resources on prevention. When criticised about this failing it claims to practice prevention, but often confuses early intervention with prevention. Why make an issue about the early detection and treatment of cancer and other chronic diseases when it is often possible to prevent them in the first place? Screening for disease is cited as an example of prevention, but often the detection of a cancer by routine screening comes too late to achieve a cure by conventional medicine. Why place emphasis upon the early detection and treatment of ischaemic heart disease when it is largely preventable by diet, supplementation, exercise and the cessation of smoking? Some screening procedures are thought to even cause cancer. Mammography is one example, especially when it is repeated annually and commenced at too an early age. This is often the case where the patient has to pay for investigation and treatment. There is the additional argument that the diagnosis can be missed, but in any event the disease may be well advanced before being capable of detection by this procedure. Other investigations are unreliable with some like the PSA (used to detect cancer of the prostate) being accurate in possibly less than 75 per cent of patients. These are examples of how governments have created a health service that is doomed to failure because of these and other omissions.

The present Government places equal emphasis upon the NHS and the educational system. However the education of both parents and children neglects the subject of health and the prevention of disease, claiming it is not within its remit. Education budgets are increasingly coming under pressure to deal with the increasing numbers of children with special educational needs that are mainly the result of preventable and treatable medical problems. Despite this, authorities will neither challenge the perceived medical wisdom nor conduct research into the causes of these various special needs problems. I know of one avenue of research that was stopped for 'political' reasons. Social services, a supposed equal partner with the NHS in the health care of communities, is far from treated as an equal partner when it comes to government funding. Consequently, although it espouses the importance of preventative measures, nearly all of the social services money has to be spent on statutory care leaving little or no money for prevention. Is this an own goal on the part of the Government or a deliberate policy of maintaining high levels of sickness?

In the absence of a coherent national program for the prevention of illness, it is not surprising that many people do not understand the need to take responsibility for their own wellbeing. Many people have been led to believe that disease and chronic ill health are both natural consequences of growing older. The idea that staggering to the late seventies and early eighties is a bonus, despite the presence of chronic illness, is a view endorsed by the medical establishment. A recent research project highlighted the fact that the last eight or nine years of life was usually spent dependent upon medicines to alleviate the symptoms of chronic ill health. Furthermore people living in the North of the United Kingdom were more at risk than those people living in the South.

The medical establishment believes these symptoms of chronic illness seldom merit a diagnosis. A patient requiring a more definite answer is told not to expect anything different at their age. In the case of a female patient there is often the added complication of being a woman as a reason for ill health. Repeated requests for a diagnosis are greeted with the view that it is all due to stress or a psychological problem. This diagnosis is rewarded with a prescription for an antidepressant or similar psychotropic drug. Stress has become a favourite excuse for unexplained ill health at any age, and because it is a word understood by everyone, patients often readily accept it, and possibly a tranquilliser as well. The present Government is now concerned that high levels of certified sickness are costing the economy too much. It has decided that stress levels are too high and that this condition forms a major percentage of all illness. It has instructed businesses and public bodies to address the cause of stress, but oddly enough there is no diagnostic test for stress. Stress represents the opinion of a doctor who is allowed by law to make a 'vague diagnosis' when he or she cannot make an accurate diagnosis. Another research project attributed the high rate of GP referral for a psychiatric opinion to a refusal to admit that they simply have no idea what to do. Study of the UK National Health Service concludes that there are more psychiatrists than GPs. There are sufficient psychologists to offer their services by having an establishment of one practitioner to serve 3 GPs. (However when it comes to diagnosing and treating serious physical medical nervous conditions there is only one neurologist for every 100 GPs!! Who is really mad?) It goes without saying that this approach brings little reward but condemns the patient to a prolonged dependency to drugs. Psychiatry rarely cures patients. Of all the symptoms neglected in this way the most prevalent is 'pathological' tiredness. There are however many natural ways in which to improve the quality of life of these elderly citizens.

In our Clinic we receive a constant stream of patients who have been condemned to persistent chronic ill health allegedly because of their age, sex or stress. Our first task is to reassure them that this is not a true reflection of their health. This news alone often lifts the burden from their shoulders. There then follows the search for the underlying cause of their illness, and then we set about treating it.

The greater an individual's fear of a specific disease, the more likely that person will seek out and follow a holistic lifestyle either to treat or to prevent it. Cancer is perceived to be the deadliest of all illnesses, although it has the same root causes as all other chronic illness, and therefore a cancer patient is more likely to strictly adhere to a particular lifestyle. Diet is the main plank of treatment and it is essential to move away from today's accepted lifestyle. For both treatment and prevention it is advised to avoid all convenience and processed foods, and the use of microwave ovens. No red meats, refined sugar, white flour, coffee, nor alcohol. The more vegetarian the diet the more alkaline the body becomes, and the less hospitable towards cancer cells. If the thought of a total vegetarian diet is unacceptable then fish and a little white meat may be added to the menu. This should be in conjunction with a high water intake. As mentioned in previous chapters, organic produce is to be preferred. This holistic approach to life offers an alternative to, or a complement to, the more traditional trio of surgery, radiotherapy and chemotherapy. In either instance this diet and other measures offers a better **quality** of life than the traditional approach which may offer little success in the treatment of cancer. It is also essential to remove any harmful chemicals from the home, which may be present in personal care and household cleaning products. All these changes to a personal lifestyle are equally important for both treatment and prevention. There are now many books offering advice upon lifestyle and diet. I can recommend "The Tree of Life" by Chris Woollams.

The above diet may be acceptable to doctors, although it may be viewed with a degree of scepticism. However the need for supplementation is more contentious. Doctors receive little or no education in nutrition yet, despite this gap in their education, many will scoff at the idea of supplementation. Today there is conflicting advice even in the field of cancer. Whilst some doctors advocate no supplements top professors at the Royal Marsden hospital give cancer patients Vitamin D and red clover. Other doctors advise patients not to take supplements during chemotherapy and radiotherapy, whereas other doctors believe that antioxidants protect healthy cells from damage during these treatments. The medical view may be correct as regards certain mineral tablets, which can pass though the intestines without any absorption of the minerals. However medical wisdom doesn't discourage the use of powerful calcium products for the treatment of osteoporosis, despite their potential to damage the intestinal tract and despite the fact that no blood calcium deficiency exists to explain the presence of osteoporosis. Osteoporosis is rarely due to oestrogen and or calcium deficiency. Deficiencies of magnesium, boron and progesterone are the more common causes of osteoporosis. The gold standard for supplementation must be Maximol (made by Neways) which is a sub-colloidal ionic suspension containing fulvic acid, a naturally occurring substance that aids absorption of the minerals and their onward transportation to the individual cells of the body. I was so impressed by the quality of Neways' products that I decided to become a distributor for the company

All animals and humans rely upon plants for their source of essential minerals. Plants have the unique ability to convert the inorganic minerals in the soil into the organic forms that are essential to sustain animal life. This conversion to an organic form and the subsequent absorption is aided by the presence of fulvic acid, which is found around the roots of plants Obviously the absence in the soil of sufficient minerals not only stunts the growth of the plant itself, but leads inevitably to the poor nutrition of both animals and humans that feed on that plant. As mentioned previously experiments with plants exposed to organic minerals and fulvic acid have shown that there is an increase in their size and nutritious goodness Supplementation with minerals and vitamins invariably leads to an improvement in the health of patients. The majority of doctors have greeted this view of the vital importance of minerals and vitamins to the health of the body with scepticism. However in my experience illness, both physical and mental, is invariably linked to one or more mineral deficiencies. Even people who think that they are fit may nevertheless have a deficiency that has yet to manifest itself in the form of disease. Anybody accepting this theory would expect to see a dramatic improvement in their health when supplementation with nutrients is added to their diet. I can understand the disappointment that may be felt after the failure to show any signs of improvement following several weeks of supplementation and lifestyle changes. At this stage a person may revert to their previous lifestyle or to explore other avenues of treatment.

For people who decide to try additional or other options there are a variety of choices. The theory of the importance of vitamin B-17 in the treatment and prevention of cancer has recently been revived. Philip Day has helped the revival of B-17 by writing and lecturing about the merits of this vitamin. Some patients who have followed this advice have made dramatic improvements, others haven't. Some patients will progress to having intravenous injections of minerals, vitamins and B-17. Although some patients will improve with the intravenous therapy, some will not, and others will fail to maintain the recovery after the treatment has been stopped. It is important to realise that no single form of treatment is the sole panacea for all forms of disease. Every person's illness is as unique as that person is also equally unique, and similarly any patient's treatment should be equally unique to that individual.

There may be several reasons why these various supplements fail to improve the health of patients. One reason for this failure to improve is due to a 'barrier' within the body that prevents the absorption of selected minerals and vitamins. Certain pathological conditions are responsible for creating these 'barriers' that in turn cause nutritional deficiencies and the subsequent symptoms and diseases that inevitably follow in their wake. The concept of a 'barrier' and the various treatments to overcome these 'barriers' will be the subject of the following chapters.

Chapter 14

The 'Barrier' Theory of Disease.
How Ill People Fail To Absorb All
Their Nutrients

There always appears to be a deficiency of one or more minerals in any chronic disease. To deny this possibility is to ignore the accepted catalogue of diseases and symptoms that are attributed to mineral deficiencies that can be found in many medical textbooks. Some of the more commonly found deficiencies and the diseases that they can cause are listed in appendix C. Research has confirmed the incidence of certain illnesses in various parts of the world where there is a proven deficiency in the staple diet (e.g. the previously mentioned high incidence of cancer in parts of China where there is a lack of selenium). Supplementation with the recommended daily intake of the missing mineral was noted to dramatically reduce the incidence of these illnesses (e.g. the noted reduction in cancer when selenium was provided in the above example of China). Studies of various populations (e.g. the Okinawans) that live to a great age, yet maintaining their health and vigour, have shown that their staple diet is rich in the complete range of essential minerals and vitamins.

However modern medicine continues to ignore nutrition's role in both prevention and treatment of disease. This arrogance is compounded by the continued failure to estimate the levels of these minerals and vitamins in the body. Measurements are however made to estimate sodium, potassium and calcium, even though any abnormal levels of these three minerals are often due to the unwanted side effects of certain medicines. Lithium is only measured to ensure that too much of this mineral is not being administered for the treatment of depression. It will be seen from the list in appendix C that lithium deficiency can lead to depression, but also to other surprisingly different and contradictory illnesses. The lack of chromium, and two other minerals, as a cause of diabetes is well known but the three minerals are seldom estimated in the specialist diabetic clinics. Selenium deficiency can also lead to a wide variety of hormonal problems, but its blood levels are never measured in the specialist hormone clinics.

The medical and national press frequently carry reports on the adverse effects upon the health of children who eat a modern diet compared with the wartime diet, despite the effects of rationing. The same comments could be made for adults. Wartime women had far fewer hormone problems and suffered less osteoporosis (even after making allowances for present day lifestyle which also contributes to osteoporosis). Poor diet due to social, financial or psychological problems is acknowledged and is used as an excuse for claiming that when eating a well balanced diet there can be no nutritional deficiency, and that supplementation is unnecessary. No one has sensibly defined a well balanced diet, nor if the desired food and how it is cooked still contains a full complement of the essential vitamins and minerals. Fit people, who supplement, rarely become stricken by chronic illness. Interesting research has been carried out in some young offenders' institutions, where consenting prisoners accepted supplements to their prison diet. These supplements were in low doses and not in the most absorbable form. However despite this, there was a remarkable improvement in their behaviour whilst in prison, and their re-offend rate when released back into the community was also much reduced. Some of this work was done specifically for the Home Office, yet has not been released for publication despite the fact that high levels of juvenile crime is now both a political and social problem. The experiment has been repeated and there was a 35 per cent improvement in the behaviour and re-offend rates, but it was decided that it was not financially viable to continue with the project. Some Juvenile Magistrates have been informed of this research but so far there have been few, if any, referrals for the estimation of nutritional status and any other underlying causes to explain criminal behaviour.

It has been mentioned in a previous chapters that a conventional medical diagnosis is of little use when it comes to identifying the actual cause of disease. Despite the drawbacks it has to be accepted that drugs will often ease the symptoms of disease.

Conversely a patient treated with nutritional supplements will often show little or no improvement. To detractors of the nutritional theory of disease, this may seem to support their opinions. They would argue that the failure of supplements to achieve any change in patients proves that minerals can play no part in disease, neither its prevention nor its cure. However because no routine blood tests are performed to measure the levels of minerals in the body, there is no proof one way or another to support the rival theories. However if a mineral shortage in the blood was found before supplements were given and if tests repeated afterwards showed no improvement, or even deterioration, then there must be a logical reason to explain it. The 'barrier' theory of illness offers a logical explanation, which is supported by the apparently successful treatment of our patients.

Ill patients appear to be incapable of absorbing one or more minerals and vitamins from their food, and any added supplements, as they pass through the stomach and intestines. If the real underlying cause for this mal-absorption could be identified and treated, then patients' health should improve as the missing nutrients can once again enter the body. Moreover there are only a few underlying conditions that can lead to a mineral deficiency. In the following chapters, six causes are identified and how they can be successfully treated. There may be other rare causes, but so far I haven't identified any. I believe that all patients like explanations for both their illness and treatment. As yet I am unable to offer a satisfactory scientific explanation for this phenomenon of mal-absorption. In addition I am unable to explain why patients exhibit only a few and not all the listed symptoms and diseases associated with any particular mineral or vitamin deficiency. Conversely if patients can identify their illness or symptoms from the list in appendix C, they can confidently predict their own mineral and vitamin deficiencies. If a patient can be so confident why can't the medical professionals be equally competent?

I try to explain to patients the 'barrier' theory and how it affects them in the following simplistic fashion. Patients are encouraged to visualise their intestines as a tube that has a number of trap doors through which the various minerals and vitamins must pass to enter into the body. Each individual mineral and vitamin has its own specific trap door, and it cannot enter into the body in any other way. The reasons why trap doors remain closed, and the keys to unlock and then open them are explained in chapters 17 to 22. The trap doors in healthy people are always open. When the trap doors of ill patients are prised open they too will begin to recover their health.

When it comes to explaining which symptoms occur with each deficiency, I like to encourage patients to think of their bodies as a tree. The trunk and roots represent the underlying cause of disease. The one two or three main branches represent the mineral deficiencies. The smaller branches, twigs and leaves growing out from these main branches represent all the various symptoms that can be caused by that particular branch's deficiency. Due to the diverse manner in which the tree grows, each small branch and its leaves have a unique structure that is different to all the other parts of that or any other tree. Another small branch taken from an adjacent part of the tree would be different from the first specimen and be equally unique. This is reflected in the uniqueness of each patient, who may share the same pathology and deficiencies of others, but nevertheless appears to have an equally unique illness. I have seen married couples, or even three or more generations of the same family, who all share the same underlying disease and deficiency, but who are either 'well', or suffering from entirely different illnesses. Following an accurate and detailed medical history I can usually predict both the deficiencies and the possible cause of the illness. It is like trying to solve a crossword puzzle. I believe that any patient should be capable of solving the puzzle of his or her own particular illness. To help anyone who is keen to solve puzzles, in Chapter 15 I will deal with the most frequently found deficiencies and in Chapter 16 I will seek to illustrate the importance of a thorough enquiry into a patient's medical history.

Chapter 15

Mineral Deficiency.
The Cause Of All Chronic Illness?

It is estimated that there are at least 67 essential minerals necessary for a long and healthy life, but that the deficiency of only a few is responsible for most chronic disease. Doctors usually confine their interest to sodium, potassium, iron and calcium. Correct blood levels of both sodium and potassium are essential for the heart's performance, and various drugs can disturb this important chemical balance. Abnormal levels of these two minerals can cause the heart to beat irregularly or even to cease beating altogether. This potentially disastrous situation explains why hospital laboratories frequently estimate the levels of these two minerals. Iron deficiency causes anaemia, and calcium is necessary for healthy bones and the correct functioning of both nerves and muscles. Calcium is also essential for the transmission of nutrients and electricity across cell membranes. Doctors routinely prescribe supplements of potassium, iron and calcium. However I very rarely discover any deficiency of sodium, potassium, iron or calcium, but this could be due to supplementation by doctors or by the patients themselves. However it could also be due to the fact that the specific 'trap doors' for these four minerals are rarely closed.

Selenium deficiency is relatively common in patients suffering from chronic diseases. Its deficiency can have the most serious consequences and is extremely dangerous because, unlike most other mineral deficiencies it can remain symptom free for months or even years. I have seen examples of men who have apparently been short of selenium since birth yet who were extremely fit and active throughout their lives but who developed cancer in their sixties and seventies. Men require less selenium than women. Therefore it takes men a longer time to use all their available selenium. Many people consider that cancer to be the most serious and dreaded illness. Selenium is invariably deficient in cases of

97

cancer. Despite this fact selenium levels are not measured in cancer patients neither do they receive any supplementation of this important mineral.

Several mainstream medical textbooks have been devoted to the role played by poor nutrition in causing cancer. Some doctors claim that a deficiency in nutrition is the commonest cause of cancer, and is therefore more important in the causation of this disease than either cigarette smoke or pollution. Lack of selenium causes impaired immunity, and therefore it is possible to assume that cancer patients are more susceptible to the effects of surgery, radiotherapy and chemotherapy. No wonder that these three procedures are poorly tolerated and have such poor results. In later chapters there will be further examples of the unfortunate outcomes due to the impaired immunity that is the result of selenium deficiency. A few consultants are now recommending some form of supplementation to boost immunity prior to courses of radiotherapy and chemotherapy. However these recommendations are for general supplements, with no specific emphasis upon the specific importance of selenium. If selenium were injected directly into a patient's veins prior to chemotherapy, radiotherapy or surgery, then the results following these three procedures could improve, despite the fact that the underlying cause of the selenium deficiency hadn't been addressed.

Women appear to be more susceptible to the effects of selenium deficiency than men. This is possible due to their endocrine system's heavier demand for this mineral. Hormones are chemical messengers that instruct various cells to perform certain functions. The pituitary gland appears to be very susceptible to the lack of this mineral. The pituitary gland produces a whole range of hormones that help to control a body's other hormone glands. For some reason not all the pituitary gland's hormones are affected, and it is possible to find only one of its hormones reduced which then compromises the function of another hormone gland. However because most of these hormone glands interact with one another it is impossible to estimate the final result if one pituitary hormone isn't produced. Therefore the ovaries, thyroid, and adrenals may be forced to produce too much or too little of one or more of their own hormones. Urinary output can also be increased in a disease called Diabetes Insipidus. It has been noted that some children taking the drug ritulin to help control their hyperactivity will not reach their anticipated height. However, because hyperactive children are often short of selenium, it is also possible that the shortage of this same mineral could also prevent the pituitary gland making its growth hormone. Several gynaecological conditions can be due to a selenium deficiency and these include infertility, polycystic ovaries, pre menstrual tension, endometriosis, irregular periods and migraine associated with a certain phase of the menstrual cycle. There has been widespread concern over the large number of hysterectomies, accompanied by the removal of ovaries. It is quite possible that many of these operations were unnecessary and could have been avoided by supplementation with selenium.

There are other heavy demands upon a mother's selenium stores. Both pregnancy and breast-feeding drain away the available minerals and vitamins from mother to her infant. This can lead to a mother becoming ill with fatigue or postnatal depression. If a mother is deficient at the commencement of the pregnancy she may miscarry or develop some other symptom of the deficiency. This is however potentially more serious to the live infant of this depleted mother. The affected baby may be premature, underweight and have a poor immune system. The defective immune system could predispose to vaccine damage (dealt with in a latter chapter) recurrent infection, or even cot death. The sudden death of an infant is not only devastating to the parents but could lead to charges of infanticide, especially if more than one child dies. If the mother who is deficient in selenium and then receives no selenium following the death of a child, then it follows that subsequent children will also be born without selenium and therefore likely to suffer a similar fate. There is no post mortem estimation of the baby's selenium, and it is unlikely mother's mineral level would be measured. If the mother is convicted and subsequently appeals against the verdict, then if at the time of that appeal her selenium is estimated and found to be grossly deficient then it is safe to assume that her dead infant was also deficient and therefore prone to cot death. In that case the cause of death should have been by natural causes, and that by not measuring selenium levels could have led to a miscarriage of justice. There is now a general concern about the safety of such convictions, but this is due to doubts about the professional judgements of the witnesses who give evidence before the court, rather than their failure to remember that deficiency of selenium is a known cause of cot death.

Selenium deficiency is usually present in the various forms of hyperactivity and those learning difficulties that are not due to physical brain damage. The numbers of these children are increasing, and placing heavy demands upon the education budgets of local authorities. Accurate figures are difficult to obtain in this country. In the USA it is estimated that 20 per cent of children with this form of disability require the provision of special educational support. Of these children, it is estimated that the incidence of autism has risen tenfold in the past few years. The presence of one mineral may cause the displacement of another, possibly toxic, mineral from the body. Selenium is known to displace mercury. Therefore in instances of autism due to vaccine damage, it is possible to postulate that a lack of selenium is responsible for a failure to eliminate from the body the mercury present in many vaccines. Estimates of the lifetime cost of an autistic patient, who is invariably deficient in selenium, in the U.K. have been put at £1,000,000, and these figures have not been disputed. Hyperactive adults usually manage to control and conceal their problem. However they are usually very active, never find time to sit down and sleep very few hours. Failure to control this disorder may lead to criminal behaviour or addiction. Alternatively these adults can suddenly become 'worn out' and end in complete fatigue, or have a medical emergency such as a heart attack. A patient who is selenium deficient may come with a history of fatigue and with no obvious history of hyperactivity.

Fatigue is a very common symptom of various deficiencies, including selenium. Failure to detect these deficiencies will leave the doctor without a definite diagnosis, and he will therefore attribute these symptoms of fatigue to stress, age, being female or just a figment of the patient's mind. Selenium deficiency is also implicated in Alzheimer's disease, Parkinson's disease, heart problems, cataracts and cirrhosis of the liver. These conditions are often attributed to the unhappy result of growing old. Should they occur at an early age the patient is considered to be very unlucky. These diseases could have been prevented or at least aided by the addition of selenium. Short term memory loss, unexplained tremors and unexplained heart palpitations can all be the result of the lack of this mineral, and the true cause of these conditions should always be suspected and treated.

The early diagnosis of multiple sclerosis is often difficult, and is finally made after several episodes of unexplained symptoms, that can appear and disappear over a period of months or even years. Muscular dystrophy is similarly difficult to diagnose in its early stages. Because the early, and diverse, symptoms are unrecognised, I believe that multiple sclerosis is far more common than is generally realised. There is always a selenium deficiency, and it is often associated with a deficiency of the fatty acid lecithin. Lecithin is an essential ingredient for the insulation of the nerve fibres. The consequences of this defective insulation of the nerve fibres are similar to the effect of poorly insulated electric cables. Therefore any minor episode of tingling, pins and needles, numbness and partial loss of sight should be treated as multiple sclerosis until proved otherwise. Effective supplementation with this mineral and the fatty acid at an early stage has a dramatic effect upon the symptoms and recovery is complete. In the latter stages of this disease the progression can be halted but complete recovery is very unlikely. It is essential to recognise that the underlying cause of the deficiencies has to be identified and treated before any successful supplementation. This emphasises the need for early diagnosis and treatment.

Another unusual feature of the deficiency of selenium is unexpectedly severe pain. Certain illnesses like shingles and migraine are associated with pain. However in the absence of selenium the severity of the patient's pain can be quite remarkable. Unfortunately the patient is then assumed to either have either a very low pain threshold, or to be overreacting. I have seen a patient with the most severe abdominal pain, who was very intensively investigated in various hospitals without a diagnosis being made, and despite this had been prescribed morphine for pain relief. I found he had a total absence of selenium. As previously mentioned selenium is also capable of displacing mercury from the body, and this may help to explain why mineral solutions, like Maximol, are so effective in treating dental patients suffering from mercury toxicity.

Magnesium is another mineral whose deficiency is a common cause of illness. Perhaps the most well known illness associated with this deficiency is ME. It was found that the deficiency was in the red blood cells; this led to the use of injections of magnesium into the buttocks or a vein. The former was very painful, and the latter time consuming and expensive. Neither procedure produced lasting relief, and this fact plus the previously mentioned inability to find a single virus responsible for the illness, fostered the belief that it was a psychological and not a physical illness. Once again, if the underlying cause for the non-absorption is identified and treated, then the patient will recover. When ME was accepted as a disease there was no suggestion given to explain the symptoms. The reality is that this illness represents another example of non-absorption that includes magnesium, and is usually caused by any virus (glandular fever virus is commonly found) or a parasite. Other less common causes include candida, vaccines, heredity or electromagnetic fields.

Some nutritionists believe that magnesium is one of the most important minerals for the proper functioning of the heart and circulation. Shortage of magnesium can be found in both low and high blood pressure. However in my experience the commonest symptom is an irregular heartbeat or palpitations. I find it difficult to persuade Cardiologists to estimate the levels of magnesium in samples of blood, especially when no other obvious pathology can be found. One patient had been admitted to hospital on more than one occasion with the consequences of an irregular heartbeat. Failure to make a diagnosis and to cure the problem led to her to be passed from one consultant physician to another. Eventually she had the courage to mention that I thought that the problem was a deficiency of magnesium. To prove that I was mistaken the consultant arranged for a blood test. A day or so latter she received an urgent call from the hospital because her blood levels of magnesium were so low. An airline pilot had his license revoked because of bouts of unexplained palpitations; again this was an example of magnesium deficiency. Another practitioner who treats airline crews tells me that palpitations in this group of patients is not uncommon.

You will see from the list in appendix C that there are a wide variety of mental symptoms associated with this deficiency. They include anxiety, anorexia, confusion, insomnia, depression, irritability, and restlessness. Of a more physical nature there are seizures, tremors and vertigo. In addition to the muscular problems of ME there may be cramps, twitching of muscles and, most commonly of all, persistent constipation.

Probably the most unsuspected consequence of this deficiency is osteoporosis. Medicine only interests itself with oestrogen and calcium. Oestrogen helps prevent the breakdown and removal of old bone. Therefore bone, which should be a vibrant tissue in which old materiel is constantly removed and then replaced by new, under the influence of oestrogen alone it will in time become brittle. That is why it is suggested that for osteoporosis HRT is of no use after 10 years. It is forgotten that progesterone is needed to manufacture new bone tissue, and patients given only oestrogen following a hysterectomy are severely disadvantaged. Doctors will have forgotten about the physiology of bone, if indeed it was part of their education, and it is not in the interests of the drug companies to remind them about this. Patients lucky, or unlucky, enough to be given synthetic progesterone will often suffer undesirable side effects. They are not offered the available and very effective natural progesterone creams because they cannot be patented and therefore of little financial advantage to the pharmaceutical companies. Those patients for whom oestrogen is contraindicated because of risk of cancer or deep vein thrombosis are then given modern strong calcium products that are known to have a high incidence of very undesirable side effects. I very rarely see osteoporotic patients that are deficient in either calcium or oestrogen. Most patients have an excess of oestrogen, despite the removal of their ovaries because other hormone glands can produce this hormone, and too there is usually an excess of oestrogen, both real and oestrogen mimics, in both food and drinking water. Patients with normal levels of calcium that are give additional calcium, will excrete any excess of this mineral by combining it with other vital minerals (like magnesium) that may already be in short supply within their bodies. It is a pity that it is not widely appreciated that for new bone tissue to be formed various other ingredients are needed, including magnesium, boron and vitamin D. Lack of these two minerals is very common in osteoporosis, and in my experience is nearly always the dominant factor. I have seen a consultant physician, who specialises in the treatment of elderly patients suffering from osteoporosis, who claimed not to have heard of boron. If this lack of knowledge regarding the importance of boron is widespread throughout the medical profession, it might help to explain why doctors have failed to protest over the present Government's agreement with the EU plans to ban boron supplements. It may also explain why there has been a very large increase in the number of patients needing orthopaedic surgery. This ignorance of human physiology will condemn thousands of people to suffer inevitable osteoporosis. Vitamin D deficiency is surprisingly not very common in the UK. However in those sunnier climates, like Australia, where there is an association between skin cancer and exposure to sunlight, it is now increasingly common to find a decrease in bone density due to Vitamin D deficiency because of the use of sun blocks and more time spent in the shade. Some doctors are now saying that the benefits of sensible sun bathing far outweigh the known risks to the skin of overexposure. For healthy bones both oestrogen and progesterone are required, plus a sensible diet with the use of carefully balanced supplements, plus the avoidance of fizzy drinks, reduction in alcohol consumption and cigarette smoking. All this plus at least twenty minutes of brisk walking (weight bearing) every day is required to maintain strong healthy bones. Some would argue that load bearing and weight bearing in the gym is more beneficial than brisk walking. However in the days when gyms were rarely available and when women walked to and from their children's schools, there was far less osteoporosis. Whatever the best preventative, it is better to walk than to drive to and from the gym in a car.

Unlike selenium, the majority of illnesses associated with the deficiency of magnesium and other minerals occur sooner rather than later. This is most marked in those cases that have initially responded to treatment and the replenishment of mineral stores, only to relapse when absorption ceases again and the body stores start to become depleted once again. There can be a sudden reappearance of symptoms like palpitations and constipation when the stores of magnesium fall. It will be seen in the next section that there can be a similar early return of symptoms in a zinc deficiency. This gives the patient a very early indication of a problem and the need to seek an early consultation with their practitioner. There are of course exceptions to every rule. Osteoporosis caused by magnesium or boron deficiency may not show itself for months or even years unless the patient is retested at an earlier date. Patients drinking a lot of milk for their osteoporosis should be aware that the calcium in milk inhibits the absorption of magnesium. Without magnesium you cannot get the calcium into the bones. Contrary to the general rule that selenium deficiency is slow to have an effect, symptoms of a recurring selenium deficiency will soon become apparent in multiple sclerosis, painful conditions and in the behavioural and learning disorders.

Zinc deficiency is associated with a long list of symptoms and illnesses. It is well known that the deficiency is associated with a loss of the senses of taste and smell. However these are relatively rare findings despite the large number of patients who lack adequate levels of the mineral. Similarly the finding of white spots on a patient's fingernails, which is supposed to be the classical symptom, is equally rarely seen. There has been some orthodox medical research into the beneficial effect of giving zinc to patients suffering from the common cold. There certainly appears to be some benefit and very many people reach for the zinc bottle at the first sign of a cold. Presumably this works by boosting the immune system, and also it is believed to help the action of vitamin C, another favourite cold remedy. Zinc can damage viral cell walls. However taking very high doses of zinc can cause cancer.

Various allergies, asthma and eczema tend to be the commonest signs of zinc deficiency. It is very rare to find an allergic condition without the coexistence of zinc deficiency. There are rare exceptions, and a baby may be born with an allergy to the likes of pork, shellfish and strawberries, which will only appear on the first occasion when these foods are eaten. Most other allergies tend to appear at a later age, or may develop slowly, and are invariably accompanied by the lack of this mineral. These symptoms tend to disappear once the cause of the deficiency is identified, treated and then followed by the replenishment of the zinc stores. A zinc-deficient infant will develop eczema at a very early age. This can be due to the mother's lack of this mineral to pass on to her offspring, or to the adverse effect of the first immunisation, usually the polio vaccine, which takes place at about 8 weeks of age. If the cause of the infant's skin condition is recognised and treated effectively rather than with the use of topical cortisone creams, the skin usually recovers and becomes free of symptoms. The return of both asthma and eczema will occur very early on when the zinc levels fall below normal, and serves to remind a patient or a carer of the need to seek further treatment.

Acne is another skin complaint associated with the lack of zinc. Brittle nails, hair loss and frizzy hair may also occur. Various mental symptoms can occur and include apathy, depression, anorexia irritability, paranoia and memory loss. A patient may experience fatigue and lethargy, but other deficiencies can also cause these problems. Pica, the cravings of pregnancy, is also associated with the lack of other minerals. Anaemia and slow healing wounds are other features sometimes found. Diarrhoea and mal-absorption are more likely to be the cause of zinc deficiency rather than the effect of an existing deficiency. Infertility and impotence can be the result of a shortage of zinc and other minerals. From the long list of possible effects due to a lack of zinc, and the consequent large number of body functions that are dependent upon the ample availability of this mineral, it is easy to realise why it is implicated in so many illnesses. Added to this there is the apparent susceptibility to the impaired absorption of this mineral in the presence of various pathological conditions.

The study of the various symptoms associated with mineral deficiency shows that there can be entirely opposite effects caused by the shortage of an individual mineral. **Lithium** deficiency is a good example of confusing and apparently contradictory symptoms. In orthodox medicine lithium tablets have been used to treat depression, although now mainly replaced by more modern drugs. However there seemed to be fewer side effects with the use of lithium, and less possibility of developing drug dependency. Lack of lithium is found in children suffering from attention deficit disorder (ADD) and hyperactivity (however these two conditions are more often associated with the lack of selenium and essential fatty acids). There can be sudden changes of mood. I have treated a young boy who could be quiet, calm and loving but would suddenly and without warning fly into a rage and lie on the floor kicking and screaming. He had punched a teacher during his first few days at school and had used a remarkably wide range of offensive language. It was difficult for his mother to reconcile the two sides of his behaviour. Treatment was effective and early signs of a relapse soon brought him back to my clinic.

Manic depression is seen where the patient swings from deep depression to a very hyperactive state. In unexplained epilepsy there is usually no attempt to measure the blood levels of lithium. I have seen a university student who developed epilepsy, due to lithium deficiency, for the first time shortly following a meningitis vaccine injection. Although not a common occurrence I have seen other epileptics with a shortage of this mineral. The occurrences of lithium deficiency are less common, and again often associated with the shortage of other minerals.

The shortages of the above four minerals in food, in association with a reduced ability to absorb them from the intestines, are commonly found in a wide variety of diseases. The inability to absorb is much less common in other minerals. However shortage of **chromium** is occasionally found. The lack of this mineral, in association with a normal pancreas, is often found in late onset diabetics, which is usually treated medically with diet and or tablets. ADD, ADHD, hyperactivity and learning disorders can also be associated with a shortage of chromium, in addition to deficiencies of other minerals and a fatty acid. Again it is worth noting how the symptoms can be complete opposites. Fatigue as opposed to hyperactivity and the high blood sugar of diabetes as opposed to low blood sugar levels.

Essential fatty acids have been mentioned several times. As their name suggest they are essential for healthy body metabolism. In appendix D there is further information on the effects of its deficiency. Our national diet is very short in these fatty acids. People living in the Mediterranean region eat far more fatty acid rich food including oily fish, olive oil and nuts. Our athletes seem more prone to injury, and this could be a reflection of the existing shortage of minerals and essential fatty acids made worse by the increased demands of excessive exercise.

There are two important things for patients to remember when receiving alternative treatment, especially when attempting to correct mineral deficiencies:

1. **Never stop taking the orthodox medication that your doctor has prescribed.**

2. **Because there can be a rapid improvement in your medical condition it is vitally important to have more frequent estimations of the various procedures that you normally undergo. This can include blood pressure readings, blood sugar and thyroid estimations. Any change should lead to a review by your doctor, possibly leading to a reduction, or even a cessation, of medication.**

I hope that you are now convinced of the importance of proper mineral nutrition not only to treat, but also to prevent illness. Despite these facts, supported by many medical publications, governments and the European Community would like to make mineral supplements unavailable to you. Can they be so uninformed, or is there another hidden agenda driven by those with a vested interest in your continued ill health? Every voice of dissent helps to persuade politicians that they are wrong. You can speculate on how great a decrease in all forms of illness that would occur if only doctors would estimate the level of minerals, and to supplement those patients found to be nutritionally deficient. Conversely if these supplements remain banned there will be an inevitable increase in all forms of illness.

Chapter 16

An Accurate Patient Medical History.
The Clues To The Cause Of Disease

"A wise man should consider that health is the greatest of human blessings, and learn how by his own thought to derive benefit from his illness"
(Hippocrates)

If you don't properly know what causes an illness, how can any doctor begin to give the correct and proper treatment. When I trained to be a doctor it was nearly four years before entering my first hospital ward and meeting my first patient. Those earlier years were spent in various academic studies including anatomy, physiology pathology and pharmacology. The study of nutrition in relation to disease was absent from our studies. It was also a requirement of my university to take a B.A. degree, which I took in animal physiology. So it was nearly four years before I knew if I would be capable of dealing with, and treating, ill people. It is therefore not surprising that a few of my colleagues chose to leave university and to use their degree to obtain other employment, or to pursue an academic career within the comfortable and familiar surroundings of the city in which they had spent the previous few years.

Today many universities have rearranged their syllabus so that almost from the first day a medical student dons a white coat and ventures onto the hospital ward. Although this means that the reality of the chosen career occurs at an earlier date, the basic academic studies are pursued in association with the start of the clinical training. There is a standard method of taking and recording a patient's medical history. Every student is expected to follow this protocol and the tutor or consultant would expect to find a written history identical to that of every other student and newly qualified doctor. There is a similar protocol for the method, order and recording of the physical examination of the patient. Once again, identical records are expected. After the first few patients this becomes rather a tedious chore, especially if the patient lacks exciting symptoms or physical findings on routine examination. In the past when patients could spend many weeks on a hospital ward, it became even more frustrating. It was rather like a soldier's training in that by repetition habits became ingrained and led to an automatic reaction when faced with a real crisis. However I don't remember being told how this routine history could provide a clue to the eventual diagnosis and treatment of a patient. I have now come to realise that an accurate history is very relevant, perhaps even more important than the many investigations that are so much a part of today's medical practice. If nothing else, an accurate medical history should reduce the number of investigations to an absolute minimum, thus saving the NHS unnecessary expense and the patient unnecessary discomfort.

With progress, promotion and experience, the patient's medical history and examination tends to become shorter and more tailored to an individual doctor's needs. This is partly due to the greatly increased workload. Patients no longer languish for many weeks in a hospital bed, a one or two-day stay being more likely. Therefore the time available per patient is reduced, and this pressure leads to a truncated and often personal approach, with a lack of detail, and even a lack of any accurate record, which in itself is often a common factor in many of the medical negligence claims. Similar pressure in general practice also leads to a reduction in the time spent doing these basic functions. With the drive towards increased specialisation in both consultant and general medical practice there has been the inevitable move towards a reduction in the scope of both the history and the examination. The holistic perspective is lost and with it the increased probability of an incorrect diagnosis and treatment. This is the very reverse of the stated aspirations for increased specialisation. In many cases specialisation is for the increased job satisfaction of the doctor rather than in the best interests of the patient. All these doctors would claim that work pressures and modern investigative techniques are valid reasons for curtailing the perceived chores of a full history and examination. We

110

should learn from the mistakes of America where the patient must choose which specialist consultant to see. I was once offered a job in America purely to advise patients on their choice of specialist consultant!

After many years of avoiding, wherever possible, these routine chores, I now find that taking a personal medical history is both exciting and rewarding. It is like solving a puzzle, but that anyone is capable of doing it, and furthermore medical qualification is unnecessary. It is worth repeating that a medical diagnosis is often unreliable, invalid or misleading. Diagnoses are often based upon the results of various tests and have no relevance to the causes of a particular disease. It is merely an aid to discover an appropriate drug for the treatment of the perceived disease. Sometimes the diagnosis means the acceptance of an illness but not its cause, for example irritable bowel syndrome or IBS really means that it is accepted that there is a problem with the function of that organ, but that the cause is unknown and that only the relief of symptoms is possible. On other occasions the physical nature of an illness is disputed and thus a mental label is attached. Other examples like menopause pre-menstrual tension and osteoporosis are unhelpful because there are various underlying causes most of which do not require hormone replacement therapy or other hormonal treatment.

When taking a history, or even attempting to make a self-diagnosis, it is only necessary to bear in mind two facts. Firstly, in all chronic illness there is a mineral deficiency. As mentioned in previous chapters the most commonly found deficiencies are one or more of magnesium, zinc, lithium and selenium. Secondly, having determined the most likely mineral deficiencies, attention should then be directed towards discovering the most likely underlying cause. There are only a very few possible pathological causes, namely parasites, viruses, fungi, vaccination damage, heredity and various forms of environmental pollution. Armed with these basic facts it is possible to make an educated guess as to an accurate diagnosis. It could for example be ME due to a magnesium deficiency following glandular fever.

The history begins with a request for the full name, address, telephone number, date of birth and occupation. This may seem

111

a rather mundane request and the age may or may not be relevant, but the address may be significant. In a family orientated practice it is not unusual to find unhealthy houses. People fall ill, die, and the new occupants suffer similar fates. Some roads or areas seem to have a significantly higher level of a variety of chronic illnesses. Some illnesses that appear to be due to living near to a nuclear plant have been well documented in the media. Less well known are the possible effects of living close to electricity pylons, electricity sub-stations, mobile phone masts or other transmitters. Some research has suggested that the type of illness may depend upon the distance away from the electrical cables of the national grid and thus the consequent strength of the resulting electromagnetic fields. Similar problems can occur when sleeping in a room with multiple electrical appliances or near to the controlling fuse box. It is not unusual to find a bedroom with an electric blanket, teas-maid, computer, radio, music station and TV. The study of clusters of childhood leukaemia has suggested that many victims live in a cul de sac adjacent to an end water main capable of concentrating a variety of possible carcinogens perhaps due to the influence of the electromagnetic fields associated with local electricity cables or electrical sub stations. People living near to a chemical plant, or to farms where the crops are sprayed, can be affected by airborne carcinogens or other toxic chemicals.

The patient's telephone number may be for a mobile phone, which should lead to questions about the amount of its use and whether it is worn, switched on, close to the body. It is possible to attach a shield to the mobile phone to reduce radiation and is the patient's phone fitted with such a device? It is equally relevant to enquire about the proximity of mobile phone masts. The place of employment carries risks. Telephone call centres are becoming more common and computers, phones (mobile or otherwise), can surround the employees. People working in chemical factories, the petroleum industry or nuclear establishments are at risk from contamination. Farm workers are becoming at greater risk with modern farming techniques that use a variety of herbicides, pesticides (including sheep dip) fertilisers, hormones and other additives.

112

After the preamble comes the enquiry about the problems that have caused the patient to seek help. This may seem straightforward, but it is often very difficult. Patients may volunteer the medical diagnosis that they have been given, but as previously stated this is of little use. However we are looking for **all** the current problems that the patient is experiencing. This should be a simple matter, but often the information has to be extracted bit by bit. This may be due the fact that most general practitioners will ration their patients to one symptom per surgery consultation. A hospital consultation can have the same consequence because, with increasing specialisation, the consultant will only require the information that applies to his particular speciality. Many relevant symptoms such as tiredness, distension, aches, pains, wind, thinning hair and weight gain will have been previously dismissed as irrelevant or a result of age or gender. Multiple unexplained symptoms may have been attributed to mental problems like anxiety, stress or depression. A patient previously labelled as neurotic by the general practitioner or consultant doesn't wish to mar a new professional relationship before their symptoms have been taken seriously. It is often difficult to explain to a patient that all the symptoms may be due to a single pathological condition, and therefore it is essential to have the full picture. Perhaps the wisest advice that I received as a medical student was to avoid making multiple diagnoses when it was possible to come to a single one. This advice came from a consultant psychiatrist who took great delight in referring back to his consultant colleagues those patients sent to him as being mentally ill, and for whom he made a physical diagnosis that had been previously missed. It has taken me many years to appreciate this advice, and only after I had realised the benefits of a holistic alternative medical approach to illness. It is very important not to accept the patient's own history without a great deal of enquiring, and even bullying. If a patient is asked if he or she thinks they know the cause of their own illness, it is surprising how often the correct diagnosis has been made and often previously rejected by other doctors.

It is important to ask the patient how long ago since they felt really well. Sometimes the answer may be years or even no recollection of feeling fully fit. Before moving onto another section of the history it is worth asking the patient if they have any ideas as to the cause of their illness. If nothing is volunteered enquire into the possibility of a bad episode of flu or even a stomach upset. Many infections of glandular fever are never diagnosed. This may be because there is an unusual set of symptoms or because some doctors refuse to believe that all age groups, and not just young adults, are susceptible to this particular virus. A stomach upset may have been the only indication of a parasitic infection, which then goes unsuspected for months or years. Recent immunisation could be relevant. The annual flu injections can cause chronic illness in a proportion of patients. People travelling to exotic countries often receive a variety of injections before they leave. Some of these patients will develop chronic symptoms before they return home. Recently returned holidaymakers may bring back more than they left with and arrive with malaria or other tropical diseases. Newer anti-malarial tablets can themselves cause a variety of illnesses, including various mental problems.

When satisfied with the current situation the next line of enquiry concerns the previous medical history. I usually start with the details of the patient's own birth. Then I ask for details of all previous illnesses, accidents and operations. This sounds simple but it is amazing how often things are forgotten and right until the end of the consultation new details will emerge. Sometimes the patient will return to mention details previously forgotten. I once sat down to write out my own past medical history, and when I reviewed the list I was surprised at what I had forgotten. When I did my list I was not under any pressure. I have had a patient who forgot to mention that she had nearly died from diphtheria. To forget meningitis or cancer is quite common and therefore enquiries must continue until the end of the appointment. When the patient has finished I will ask about tonsils, adenoids and appendix. Also I would like to exclude jaundice and glandular fever. I will ask about immunisations and trips to other countries. If there are household pets, especially if they are made a fuss of, I will look for parasites. I always enquire about alcohol consumption. I am not interested in its social context but whether they have become intolerant to alcohol. A significant number of parasites excrete alcohol that can cause a variety of problems that will be discussed in Chapter 18 devoted to parasitic infections.

It is then necessary to explore the family history. The health of parents, or if deceased their causes of death, may be relevant especially if there had been a significant chronic disease. Quite often the parents may be described as being well, but under pressure of questioning a whole list of chronic problems may emerge that had been dismissed as insignificant. Many people have been conditioned to believe that chronic ill health is the norm, and an inevitable consequence of life and that long-term medication will keep them alive and functioning. It may even be necessary to enquire about the health of both sets of grandparents. The health of both brothers and sisters is important, as is the health of the patient's own children. The total family history is important if there is a hint of hereditary disease. If there is a hereditary factor then it may be equally important to treat the patient's own children. If there is a significant family history of tuberculosis, cancer, diabetes, rheumatoid arthritis, pernicious anaemia, dementia multiple sclerosis or similar significant illness, then hereditary factors are more likely. However it is important to stress to the patient that it is not necessarily the disease that is inherited, but merely the inability to absorb all their nutrition. It is possible to have three generations of the same family present in the clinic, all with the same deficiencies, but each presenting with a different illness.

Female patients are asked about the various aspects of their menstrual life. "When did their periods start?" and, if relevant, "when did they cease?" "Were they regular, heavy, painful or leading to flooding and clotting?" "Were there any premenstrual symptoms, if so what sort, how severe and did the rest of the family threaten to leave home?" This is the time to enquire about any gynaecological diagnoses that had been made and if there had been any use of oral contraceptives or HRT. If there had been a hysterectomy, "were the ovaries removed at the same time and what reason was given for advising an operation?" Many women do not know why they had to have a hysterectomy! Often the use

of hormones is unnecessary, especially if there had been successful pregnancies. Any apparent hormonal imbalance in these
circumstances is likely to be due to a mineral deficiency affecting
the pituitary or other gland, or even the use of too much oestrogen medication. Selenium deficiency is the commonest cause of
hormonal problems. The age, sex, health and birth details for all
the children are important. The ease of conception will give clues
as to the fertility of both partners. "Have there been any sponta-
neous miscarriages or even terminations of pregnancy?" All these
questions may throw light upon a possible cause of the mineral
deficiency. Never forget to ask a man about the health of any
children that he has helped to conceive.

Always in need of more information, I then proceed to ask
about more specific parts of the body. This often produces some
piece of information that had previously been omitted. This
starts with head enquiring about sight, hearing, headaches and
the teeth. If there is hay fever then I think of zinc deficiency. Is
there tinnitus for which there are many explanations. If
headaches are a problem this may be the first mention of
migraine and in my mind that raises the prospect of a selenium
deficiency.

The question, "are you chesty?" may elicit the first mention of
asthma or bronchitis. The information that colds often lead to
chesty symptoms is very common. How many courses of antibiotics have there been for chest or other infections? "Does the
patient smoke or had done so in the past?" In female patients I
then enquire about their breasts. I am amazed at how often the
patient will then mention for the first time a previous removal of
a cancer or a benign lump. Multiple benign breast lumps and
cysts suggest lack of selenium and progesterone. Even a 'successful' removal of a breast cancer suggests to me that selenium deficiency is probably still present, and even though the patient feels
that they have been cured, in reality they will still be prone to
further cancer or other chronic diseases. "Do you know anything
about your heart and blood pressure?" will often produce a
history of heart attack, angina, raised cholesterol, treatment of
raised blood pressure and palpitations. Always think of possible
reasons for these conditions. Often when the blood pressure is

mentioned the female patient may volunteer that she had toxaemia in pregnancy, and this despite the fact that the various pregnancies had been previously questioned and described as normal.

I then enquire about the state of the stomach to see if there are any foods that cause problems or if there is any pain distension or wind. "Is there constipation, diarrhoea or even the one following the other on a regular basis?" I enquire about any previous diagnosis of IBS, hiatus hernia or of any stomach upset that had occurred especially when abroad. Vegetarians may be more prone to parasitic infection because of the greater quantities of fruit and vegetables they consume, especially if eaten uncooked, unwashed or unpeeled. Organic food whilst being free of herbicides and pesticides is more likely to contain parasites. An admission of a sweet tooth raises the probability of a shortage of chromium.

Next I enquire about the urinary system. I wish to know how often urine is passed, in what volume and if any pain accompanies it. "Is sleep disturbed by the frequent desire to visit the toilet?" "Have there been any infections of the bladder or kidneys, and if so what type of infection and how often did they occur and were antibiotics prescribed?" It is astonishing how often antibiotics are given before there is proof of infection. On many occasions there is no attempt to even prove that there is an infection or even to confirm that the urine is clear and free from infection following a course of antibiotics. The problem is that very few people are willing to wait for the laboratory test to be completed before starting treatment. This raises several queries. "Has the use of antibiotics caused an overgrowth of candida, or has the presence of vaginal candidiasis itself been mistaken for urinary infection?" "Could the patient have forgotten to mention the existence of vaginal candida, or volunteered that there is abdominal distension, wind, pain and food intolerances associated with the overgrowth of candida within the bowel itself?" The presence of parasitic infection can often lead to symptoms of urinary infection, and is more often the cause of both 'urinary infection' and 'candida'.

Next I turn my attention to the state of the bony skeleton. The patient may have forgotten to mention previous bone fractures. Aching bones may signal the presence of unsuspected osteoporosis. Joint pain may too be due to osteoporosis and not osteoarthritis. It is amazing how often patients believe and accept that aches and pains are a normal process of advancing age, and therefore not worthy of any mention. Painful, hot and swollen joints should not be dismissed as an infection or some local acute arthritis. It is wise to consider that the symptoms may be caused by the mal-absorption of minerals, usually selenium, and therefore the reason for the mal-absorption should be sought. In fibromyalgia and ME the pain may be in muscle rather than in bone. Nerve pain can be confused with joint pain, especially in the hip and knee joint areas. A history of back pains should be considered as a clue that nerve pain could mimic joint pain. Conversely an unsuspected joint problem could be wrongly considered to be a nerve or back problem.

Sleep is a favourite topic for discussion, and could provide vital clues to the true underlying cause of the problem. "I could sleep for England". "I sleep for hours but wake exhausted". "I fall asleep after lunch". "I cannot get off to sleep". "I wake very early and then I cannot go to sleep again". "My sleep is very disturbed". These are all very common remarks. Any pain or the frequent needs to pass urine are obvious causes of sleep disturbance. If these are successfully treated then normal sleep patterns should be restored. If the mind is still very active even when the body is exhausted, then there could be hyperactivity due the absence of selenium, chromium or essential fatty acids. This is far easier to spot in children who exhibit hyperactive tendencies during the day. However it may be more difficult to spot in adults who have successfully hidden their hyperactivity and channelled their efforts into, "never sitting down and always being on the go". These adults will try to persuade you that their problems are all due to worry and stress. It is important to realise that long-term hyperactivity will eventually lead to exhaustion, especially in adults. Therefore in those adults appearing to be exhausted it is important to discover any history of previous hyperactivity, even as far back in time as early childhood.

Classical homoeopaths have to rely very heavily upon a full

personal history and their reference books. They will explore the personal medical history in far greater detail and proceed to additional topics. In addition to enquiries about sleep, they will enquire about dreams. Different dreams or phobias may suggest different homoeopathic remedies. However, vivid dreams could signal hyperactivity, infestation with parasites, or even the side effect of prescription or recreational drugs. The effects upon the patient of various weather conditions will be explored. They are particularly interested in any unusual features including the effects of hot and cold weather. "Are there any unusual effects of high winds, thunder or other unusual weather features?" " Does any particular time of day or night hold any unusual features of patient behaviour?" Homoeopaths will delve into a patient's character. "Are they introverts or extroverts, tidy, untidy or a perfectionist?" " Does the patient like music, dancing, travel and the sea?" "Can they be happy in their own company and are there any unprovoked sudden swings in behaviour?" "How tactile are they?" The total pattern of these various personal traits can determine the final selection of a particular homoeopathic remedy. I still rely upon a shortened homoeopathic history because although I tend to rely upon the more modern and powerful resonance homoeopathic remedies, I still have recourse to use the classical remedies.

If, like me, you enjoy solving puzzles and crosswords, you should enjoy making an educated guess as to the cause of an illness when you have conducted a thorough medical and personal history. I am fortunate enough to have had a medical training to help me attempt to solve the puzzle posed by a particular illness. However you too can solve the puzzle once you have read chapters 18 to 23.

Chapter 17

My Personal Choice Of
Tools And Treatments

There is one straightforward machine I use, that if provided in all doctor's practices tomorrow and the doctors and nurses trained to use it, would cut waiting times and illness in half. It can help diagnose the cause of illness. It is widely used in Germany, and rarely in the UK. This is perhaps why other countries envy the German system of medicine. Other practitioners may use entirely different equipment, techniques and treatments. However many of these machines and treatments rely upon measuring the differing energies in the various parts of the human body. The Germans and others on the continent often refer to this practice as functional medicine. In other words, is the body functioning normally, or simply under performing? Somebody with a severe hangover may feel like dying, but experience tells him or her that they will recover. I use this extreme analogy to demonstrate to patients that many of their own symptoms are the result of their body's underperformance. In orthodox medicine the word 'functional' is used to describe a condition that is imagined rather than being a physically recognisable illness. That is the vital difference between the two types of medicine. Orthodox medicine only recognises proven disease as opposed to all the other conditions that may have no proven disease or diagnosis. Functional medicine, to alternative practitioners, recognises three conditions: Namely perfect health, proven disease, and a third larger group of people who are not functioning properly and cannot be classified as either well or ill.

Vega of Germany makes our main piece of equipment. There are several different models available and we have chosen the Vega 'expert'. This current updated computer model has a very extensive range of tests for both diagnoses and treatments. It is based upon electrical measurements of energy between two points and the patient holds a baton in one hand and a measuring stylus completes the circuit when applied to the palm of the opposite hand or to the foot. *(More information can be obtained from the U.K importers, Noma (Complex Homoeopathy) ltd., Unit 3, 1-16, Hollybrook Road, Southampton. SO16 6RB). In England this machine does not receive the recognition that it deserves; worse, efforts have been made to discredit it. Several documentary programmes have depicted non-professional, untrained people using earlier types of this machine with consequently poor results. Despite promises made by the TV production teams neither medical practitioners trained in the use of these machines or representatives of the manufacturer were called upon to allow a balanced debate. However Vega is known throughout the world as a manufacturer of high quality measuring instruments. Some time ago there were in excess of 14,000 of the Vega 'expert' machines in German doctors' and dentists' surgeries. It is important to understand that many orthodox practitioners in Germany accept the test results obtained by this machine. Legal requirements in Germany allow for an alternative medical opinion if traditional medicine fails to resolve an illness and as a consequence many German doctors practice both orthodox and alternative medicine. German dentists too find it a very useful piece of equipment, and many dentists are also qualified in medicine. Like all equipment it is only as good as the operator. Anyone can buy a stethoscope to make them look like a doctor, but it takes many years of practice as a doctor to become capable of identifying all the different sounds that the human heart can make in both disease and health. The same situation applies to the use of the Vega machines, and because many of the measurements made are qualitative and not quantitative, it requires training and practice to ensure a meaningful diagnosis and subsequent treatment. In the right hands the machine is an excellent medical tool. In orthodox medicine it could, and possibly should, be used for an initial screening and the results of which could then be confirmed by orthodox investigations. This would preclude much wasted time and expense whilst sparing patients unnecessary inconvenience.

Treatment normally comprises the use of one or more different therapies. The mainstay of our practice treatment, although I am

121

a fully qualified orthodox doctor, is homoeopathy. A German, Dr. Samuel Hahnemann, who was born in 1755, is credited with the introduction of homoeopathy. Like so many physicians of that era, he had other talents including a scientific background and the knowledge of several languages that enabled him to translate scientific articles that had been published in a variety of other countries. This ability to translate scientific literature not only helped to support him financially during his earlier years, but also may have given him certain clues that he eventually used to formulate his theory for the treatment of disease that is now known as homoeopathy. We do know that he carried out numerous experiments upon his family and his students that expanded his knowledge of homoeopathy. We also know that his treatment of patients using homoeopathy was very successful, frequently achieving better results than the conventional medicine of that time.

This form of homoeopathy has become to be known as **classical** homoeopathy. It is this form of homoeopathy that is taught and used in the homoeopathic hospitals, and the various educational institutions that train non-medical practitioners. It involves the choice of a single homoeopathic remedy that is determined following a detailed history of the patient and the study of various reference books that describe the various properties of remedies and the symptoms that they will help to treat. Various continental countries too have a tradition of homoeopathic practice, but they have progressed Hahnemann's ideas further. The first change involved mixing various remedies to form **complex** homoeopathic remedies. The true reason for the use of this type of treatment is debateable. It may be that there is a synergistic reaction between the various ingredients that leads to a more powerful effect than the use of single remedies. Cynics will argue that it is a form of cheating in that the use of a 'shot gun' approach is intellectually inferior to the original method of working out the correct remedy in the manner briefly described above. Another difference is that now many continental homoeopaths use a different system of manufacturing the remedies.

New technology is used to produce the third generation of

treatments known as **resonance** homoeopathy. Various doctors, including Dr. Helmut Schimmel and Dr. Roy Martina, have pioneered this particular branch of homoeopathy. For readers with knowledge of both physics and homoeopathy, the following quotes attributed to Dr. Martina may be helpful:

> "Each living tissue has its own specific resonance or vibration. In a state of disease this resonance is disturbed and is no longer in harmony with the rest of the body. By introducing specific resonances that will amplify an organ's natural harmonic resonances the therapy will result in less stress and more energy directed towards healing"

> "When ingredients are mixed over a certain potency range and are succussed (a traditional method of shaking together various ingredients to produce a specific homoeopathic remedy), a new frequency is created with its own energetic signature or characteristics. In other words, the remedy, despite having several ingredients, acts as one synergistic remedy."

Thus this involves the use of physics to calculate the effects of different remedies in different strengths designed to perform specific tasks. As the name implies it achieves its effect by resonance. This can be used in a variety of ways, not only to destroy infecting organisms including viruses, but also to restore the normal energy function of various parts of the body. This has created a range of powerful substances that work, in some cases where there are no pharmalogical equivalents, in safety and devoid of the many serious side effects that are associated with the use of conventional drugs. In subsequent chapters there are descriptions of how these resonance homoeopathic remedies can be used to treat those conditions that conventional medicine is unable help.

I realise that a great deal of energy has been used to denigrate the practice of homoeopathy, and for that matter other alternative treatments. I feel that this is partly due to the threat it poses to the pharmaceutical industry that plays such a major role in modern medicine. For those people who have witnessed its effectiveness and safety there can be no doubt that it is the basis of successful treatment. Physicists are able to calculate the effects of both treatment and prolonged use. They can also calculate the strengths and combinations of remedies that are required to achieve a specific therapeutic effect. The implosion theory of water, described in a previous chapter, adequately explains a possible explanation of how homoeopathy works. I also understand that some religious sects believe that it is satanic witchcraft. However it is a very brave or bigoted person who refuses to try this form of treatment when all other forms of treatment have failed. However it is always possible to die in ignorance.

As the practice of traditional medicine is failing in such a spectacular manner we can expect the attacks to become more vitriolic. Various Governments and the EU will no doubt support these attacks that appear to have originated from the pharmaceutical industry. Surely the main reason is the conflict between health and the pharmaceutical industry profits. This may be compounded by ignorance and by poor, and even biased, advice. As I mentioned before there is however the more sinister view that ruling politicians have a vested interest in perpetuating avoidable chronic illness, not only to reduce the size of populations, but also to reduce the pension burden by shortening life expectancy. Whatever the reasons, the British Government still maintains homoeopathic hospitals within the NHS.

There appear to be three reasons why homoeopathy is attacked:

Firstly, trials of effectiveness cannot be carried out in the same way as conventional drugs. Conventional drugs are designed to reduce the symptoms of specific conditions, and therefore it is relatively easy to compare one drug against another in any diagnosed medical condition. Drugs are often licensed for use in specific medical conditions. However the same homoeopathic remedies can be used in a wide variety of different illnesses, and more importantly different patients need different remedies despite sharing the same specific diagnosis and symptoms. Drugs are usually manufactured in relatively few dosages, whereas there are limitless numbers of different strengths for each individual homoeopathic remedy. Of equal importance in the effectiveness of a homoeopathic remedy is its actual strength. A drug may still work even in a dose that is either too low or too high. However it is not unusual to find that a homoeopathic remedy can only work in a specific strength. This complicates the job of a homoeopath unless there is access to a machine like the Vega 'expert' that can not only confirm the choice of remedy, but also the correct dose and how often it is needed. This is why the relative effectiveness of homoeopathy is not capable of being compared to drugs by using the same protocols that are used in pharmacology. It is obvious that to compare one homoeopathic remedy in a single specific strength against a pharmaceutical product in the treatment of a specific illness is a pointless exercise. However an article in a medical journal did admit that, in the treatment of illness, a specifically chosen remedy in a correct strength could be effective.

Secondly, orthodox medicine is unhappy that there are no trials to determine the toxic or lethal effects of homoeopathic remedies. This fails to understand the non-toxic nature of these remedies. Arsenic is well known to be a very poisonous substance that has often been used to kill people. This knowledge may cause alarm when offering a patient a homoeopathic preparation made from arsenic. The homoeopathic arsenic has been diluted and treated so many times that no molecule of this metal is still present. However the chemical has left its energetic print in the solvent that becomes the active medicine. *(Again refer to the water implosion theories in a previous chapter). Homoeopathic arsenic is a very effective remedy, but that it is no longer capable of harming people An additional safety feature is that it is possible to swallow or suck a whole supply of a remedy at a single time, but that the effect of this is no different to taking a single tablet. The same cannot be said when swallowing a whole bottle of medicines. Despite the safety feature this doesn't fail to stop the regulatory bodies banning homoeopathic or herbal remedies at the mere suggestion of one or two reported adverse effects. Some countries will even ban certain specific strengths of a particular remedy. This is in marked contrast to the treatment of pharmaceutical products that are rarely banned despite known toxic effects, plus numerous reported adverse events including the death of patients.

Finally, there have been efforts to disprove the theoretical and factual evidence that water has a memory. This phenomenon has been described in this and a previous chapter. To accept this theory destroys any counter argument that because homoeopathic remedies are so dilute, and that because there are no original molecules left, there can be no therapeutic effect. Of course, this is a huge issue with many vested interests beyond the homoeopathy 'bashers'. There are potential implications for a whole variety of industries if in fact water has a memory for harmful chemicals and can therefore exert adverse effects even after they have been removed from the water. Additional support for the theory of water quality and its memory comes from the work of a Japanese Doctor Masaru Emoto. He has photographed ice crystals of water obtained from a variety of sources and which had been exposed to many different chemical substances. He has found that these specimens of water that had been exposed to different chemicals of different strengths and in different combinations all produced different shaped crystals. His book, 'Messages from Water', contains many colour photographs to illustrate the text. *(This book is available from, The Spiral of Tranquility, PO 3747, Weymouth, Dorset. DT3 5YD : Tel. 01305816644.)

We also use a range of **herbal** remedies. Herbal medicine has been practiced for many hundreds, possibly thousands, of years. Herbalists often mix their own remedies from a selection of original tinctures. However, in general, we use mixtures, in tablet or capsule form that have been manufactured under strict factory conditions. We do however use some manufactured liquid and cream products. These can be used in a variety of ways. The remedies can include potent killers of parasites, or boosters of the immune system, boosters of physical performance, or supporters or regulators of a whole variety of bodily functions. These herbal

126

remedies can either be used alone or in combination with other therapies. In general, alternative remedies can be used safely in conjunction with conventional medicines. **However it must be noted that some herbal remedies should not be used in conjunction with certain medicines and these unacceptable interactions have been well documented in various textbooks that are available to both the medical profession an to alternative medical practitioners.**

Most people will be acquainted with **Bach flower** remedies, and especially the "rescue remedy". Today there is a diverse range of similar remedies from all over the world. They have many different applications, mostly for treating physical conditions as opposed to the mental applications of Bach flower remedies. Although we may use them for any of their known uses, they are more likely to be used to treat or prevent parasitic, viral or fungal infections. The other important use is to help restore diseased cells to their normal function. Although not strictly flower essence remedies, we also use a comparatively new range of products called **Phytobiophysics**, the result of the work by Professor Dianna Mossop who is based in Jersey. These remedies can be used on their own to treat a whole range of illnesses. They appear to work in a similar manner to homoeopathy, and so we use them not only on their own but, more frequently, in combination with homoeopathic remedies. Used in this combination there appears to be synergy that permits the homoeopathic remedy to work far longer than would be anticipated using only homoeopathy. This range of treatments also includes alternatives to routine immunisations, including the contemporary threats like anthrax or smallpox. Like homoeopathic remedies they may also be used to reverse the adverse effects of formal immunisation.

Magnetism and its therapeutic applications are likely to have an increasing role in the prevention and treatment of disease. Treatment with magnets has been practiced for thousands of years. Interest in this subject intensified following the discovery that early astronauts suffered ill effects when deprived of the normal earth's magnetic fields. Prior to the manned exploration of space the study of magnetism and magnetic fields was mainly confined to the physics laboratories. This unexpected effect upon astronauts generated a renewed interest in magnetism and to the production of various pieces of equipment designed to protect astronauts. Several companies then proceeded to use these advances in knowledge of the relationship between health and magnetism to manufacture a variety of products. The largest provider of these products is the Japanese company Nikken. Their range of products includes magnetic mattresses, overlays, pillows, back supports, portable treatment mattresses, belts, wrist straps, credit card shaped magnets designed to fit into pockets and a variety of magnetic rollers for body massage. They used to produce a portable, battery driven, electromagnetic machine also capable of fitting into a pocket. Another by-product of the space programme was the manufacture of photon discs. Photons are units of solar energy and when strapped to the skin photon discs are very powerful pain relievers, and promoters of healing.

Nikken and other companies made a variety of medical claims. However despite the widespread use of these various magnetic devices, and their apparent effectiveness, very few doctors took an interest in this subject. In the relief of pain they are generally effective. It was noticed that lying upon the magnetic mattress produced an increase in the production of urine. Many people wear magnetic products to protect them from the harmful effects of electromagnetic radiation that are present in their environment. Magnets used by astronauts to combat the effects of reduced gravity, must help to protect them from all the other radiations that are present in space. Although some doubts may persist, if a patient's health improves accompanied by a return to nutritional normality there must be some reason in the absence of other treatments. People suffering from angina claim relief of pain when wearing the credit card shaped magnet over their heart. This assumes that the magnet affects the iron in the red blood cell which, when becoming magnetised itself, then repels other red cells and by discouraging clumping allows freer passage though the narrowed coronary arteries. An indirect benefit to health comes from placing magnets around the fuel supply pipes to various engines. There is an improved fuel consumption that can have financial as well as environmental benefits. Good news to individuals, but probably not so to the energy producers and their shareholders.

I cannot explain why so few doctors have taken an interest in the medical application of magnetism, apart from its use in various diagnostic machines like the MRI scanner. However an American, Dr. William H Philpott, has written a very good book describing his experiences in the use of magnets. I can recommend this book, 'Biomagnetic Handbook', available in the UK by telephoning 01372 456287. In fewer than 100 pages he manages to impart a lot of information in a very easily understood form. This ranges from the theory of magnetic poles and their magnetic fields, to a description of various magnets, their strengths, and their various uses in medicine. Dr Philpott describes how he treats a wide range of both mental and physical illnesses. He cautions against the use of strong magnets, especially positive magnetic energy, except under medical supervision. He also describes how magnets can be used to protect the body against hazardous electromagnetic interference. Other uses include treating water and counteracting jet lag. If further reading about magnetism is required then I can recommend "Discovery of Magnetic Health" by George Washnis and Richard Hricak.

One important medical use of magnets is in the treatment of osteoporosis and the associated increased rate of healing bone fractures. Fractures exposed to magnetic fields can unite in about three quarters of the time normally expected. This is one area of magnetic medicine where other doctors have carried out research. Orthopaedic Surgeons have confirmed this accelerated healing, especially when electromagnets are inserted into the plaster of paris casts. Despite the demonstrated successes there was been no widespread use of magnets in the treatment of bone fractures

We are interested in the possible benefits of magnetic treatment. However we only use them for the treatment of pain. We use rotating magnets fixed into rollers. The patient can use small rollers, but the larger rollers, usually used to treat the back, obviously need another person to apply the treatment. Small rollers can be used for a variety of conditions including migraine and various locally painful conditions. Sometimes if the patient's pain is localised to a small area we may fix a small magnet to that spot with adhesive plaster.

We also use **acupuncture** for pain relief, especially for back and knee joints. Acupuncture has been practiced for thousands of years. It is an important part of the Chinese medical culture and has been refined over the years. The Chinese concept of disease is very different to that of modern Western medicine. Chinese doctors measure twelve pulses to our single one, and they take a keen interest in the condition of a patient's tongue. They believe that energy flows though the body in well defined channels called meridians. These meridians have certain points along their length where acupuncture needles are inserted. Neither the meridians nor the acupuncture points have been demonstrated by anatomical dissection, but certain photographic procedures have highlighted spots that correspond to the acupuncture points. There have been reports of using radioactive substances that have accumulated in greater densities at the known acupuncture sites. The Chinese believe that two sorts of energy, yin and yang, flow through these channels and that in health the two should be balanced. Conversely ill health is due to an imbalance, and the aim of acupuncture is to achieve rebalance. I find it difficult to think like a Chinese doctor, and so I confine my acupuncture to the relief of pain as described above. Various NHS acupuncture clinics have been established to treat pain.

As an introduction to acupuncture I can recommend "Modern Chinese Acupuncture" by G Lewith and N Lewith. This husband and wife team spent some time in China studying the traditional Chinese methods of acupuncture. For those people who would like to pursue an interest in acupuncture without the use of needles there are two other possibilities. Firstly there is electro-acupuncture and there are several models on the market. These models usually come complete with a guidebook for their various medical applications. Finally there is acupressure where the operator uses finger pressure rather than needles. This is useful when treating nausea and seasickness. The operator uses pressure over the front of the forearm, in the mid-line about $1/2$ of an inch above the skin crease. My wife will testify to the effectiveness of this particular treatment, especially when there are no available needles. Dr Julian Kenyon has written a good book describing the use of acupressure.

Although I do not use acupuncture for the treatment of other medical conditions, I am not disadvantaged because the Vega expert machine works on the same principles of energy and meridians. It can measure yang and yin, and the object of treatment is to restore energy balance allowing the body to help heal itself. The machine even contains a test that allows an operator to decide whether or not acupuncture will help the patient.

Aromatherapy oils are occasionally recommended, but we ourselves do not perform massage. Some continental hospitals use aromatherapy oils for reasons other than massage, and this can include lavender oil for healing burns or to combat airborne infections.

Lastly, and probably most importantly, we rely upon a range of highly effective **nutritional** products. Because lack of nutrition appears to be responsible for all chronic illness, it is vitally important to have an effective range of products to use either alone or in conjunction with other treatments. These same products are essential to prevent illness, and also to maintain good health following successful treatment of illness. Consequently we use a product that contains essential minerals in a sub-colloidal ionic and positively charged state plus essential vitamins and amino acids. This product is called Maximol and is marketed by Neways. More importantly this liquid also contains a product called fulvic acid. This substance, which is naturally occurring and essential to plant life, aids the absorption of nutriments from the bowel. However it also transports these nutrients to individual cells and then leaves the cells carrying waste products that it carries and disposes of into the bowel. Horticultural experiments have shown that if fulvic acid is applied to selected areas of land, then plants within that area grow much more vigorously than identical plants grown in an adjacent plot.

In today's hostile environment, antioxidants are essential to maintain good health. Substances called free radicals attack the body. These are normally occurring by-products of metabolism that can attack and damage various parts of the body, and nowadays we produce even more free radicals and more such toxins invade us. Antioxidants neutralise free radicals and because of the lack of these substances in our diet and an inability to make them in the body, it is wise to supplement with antioxidants. The two antioxidants mixtures that I use are revenol and cascading revenol, both produced by Neways.

However just prior to the publication of this book I learnt of yet another antioxidant, which is probably the most powerful at present available to us. It is marketed in the form of a fruit juice made from the whole fruit of a tropical tree called the Mangosteen, which is thought to have originated in Thailand. The juice has an ORAC value (oxygen radical absorbance capacity) of between 17,000 and 24,000. Its strength and uses are mainly due to the presence of a number of phytonutrients called xanthones. Xanthones are chiefly found in the pericarp (peel) and hence the need to include the whole fruit in the juice. Various ingredients of the fruit, but mainly the xanthones, have been extensively studied in many independent laboratories throughout the world. These research projects have confirmed many of the folklore benefits claimed for this fruit. The researches have suggested that there may be many potential benefits of using this fruit in the treatment of many chronic diseases. However its most important long-term benefit may lie in the prevention of disease.

An American company decided to produce a fruit juice as a result of studying the published research material on both mangosteen and xanthones. The company and its product are both called Xango. Although this juice has only been available for about two years there is already a great deal of anecdotal clinical evidence to suggest that the results of using the juice justify both the research and folklore claims. Some American doctors have found that they can substitute the juice for conventional medicines. It can also be effectively used in combination with some conventional medicines. It has a powerful anti-inflammatory action and it has arrived on the market at a time when there are questions regarding the safety of many conventional anti-inflammatory drugs. It is also a potent pain killer. If you are interested in discovering more information on xanthones and mangosteen then vist www.pubmed.com

I have had very little time to fully evaluate its benefits, but so far I have witnessed many exciting outcomes that tend to confirm the many claims that have been made about this product. It may appear to be all too good to be true. However several prominent researchers into mangosteen and xanthones have been hired by major pharmaceutical companies anxious to develop new and safer products for the treatment of disease. I am convinced that in the months and years ahead we will hear much more about this fruit and it uses.

The third group of important nutrients vital for good health are the essential fatty acids, which despite their importance are rarely found in sufficient amounts in today's western diet. Like vitamins essential fatty acids cannot be produced by the body and therefore must be part of the diet. There are a variety of fish and other oils available and it is important to take both omega 3 and omega 6. There is the ever-popular evening primrose oil, and more people seem to be using flax seed oil. They are an essential ingredient in the make up of cell membranes and therefore play a vital role in the function of cells. They are also an essential ingredient for the manufacture of several important chemicals that a healthy body must make. Athletes and people doing heavy manual labour require additional essential fatty acids.

So what diet is recommended? Firstly a reduction in red meats, alcohol, coffee, milk and refined products like white flour and sugar. Dispense with convenience foods and microwave cookers. Incline towards a vegetarian diet that in turn tends towards a more alkaline body that is more hostile to the development of chronic diseases like cancer. Wherever possible choose organic produce that is free from toxic herbicides and pesticides. However the word organic doesn't necessarily mean that there is a full complement of minerals vitamins enzymes and essential fatty acids. Choose fish and white meat; again try to avoid products contaminated by chemicals and industrial pollutants. Finally never underestimate the importance of drinking plenty of clean water. It may become increasingly important to consider the installation of good quality water filters. Reverse osmosis is reputed to be the best filter. It is increasingly important to filter out parasites from our tap water, and reverse osmosis does this too.

Chapter 18

Parasites: The Great Medical Deception

Diseases caused by parasites have now reached epidemic proportions, but doctors fail to diagnoses and treat them. It is a scandal that so many people have been left undiagnosed and untreated with nothing more than drugs to relieve their chronic symptoms.

Patients expect to be given a diagnosis. But they have become used to having a vague diagnosis, for example being told that they have a "viral illness", but not being told the specific name of the virus.

However, they certainly do not expect to be told that they are hosting a parasite, because parasites are neither suspected nor looked for during conventional medical practice. Tell someone they have a parasite though, and it is impossible to predict their reaction. Some patients will react badly and assume that you think that they have been accused of having dirty habits. "Please don't tell my family and friends that I have a parasite", is a common request. However many other patients are relieved because at long last they have an explanation for their various symptoms. One such patient was so relieved that when he had been cured of a longstanding health problem he scoured the professional microbiology and parasitology literature for any reference to diseases caused by parasites. He then wrote an article for an alternative medical magazine detailing the results of his research. Unfortunately I have misplaced the article and the name of the author. I did however cut out the following list of diseases (slightly modified by me) that was printed at the end of his article. Every single disease listed had been found in a medical publication, and had been directly linked to a parasitic infection.

I now give the following list to every patient after I have made the diagnosis of parasitic infection. The list is NOT exhaustive and I believe that parasites can cause any of illnesses that affect mankind.

Abdominal pain	Hepatitis	Thrush
Allergy	High blood pressure	Urinary infection
Alzheimers	Hyperactivity (ADD)	Urethritis
Anaemia	Impetigo (skin infections)	Urticaria
Anorexia	Irregular heart beats	Warts
Arthritis	Irritable bowel syndrome	Weight gain
Bloating	Mental confusion	Weight loss
Cancer	Migraine	Vascular changes
Chronic fatigue	Mouth ulcers	
Conjunctivitis	Myalgia	
Cystitis	Nervousness	
Depression	Oedema	
Dermatitis	Osteomyelitis	
Eczema	Personality change	
Epilepsy	Rheumatic fever	
Headache	Sore throats	

Cancer was the notable omission from the original list, and there-fore I have added it. Many cancer patients have parasites, a sele-nium deficiency and excess alcohol in their bodies. Some practitioners believe that parasites are always present in cancer patients. However I believe that it is a mistake to attribute the cause of any disease, and that includes cancer, to any single pathological process. Dr Hulda Clark is convinced that parasitic infestation is present in cancer patients and must be treated in any program that tackles the cancer. Although viruses and fungi are also technically parasitic in their behaviour, they are dealt with separately in following chapters. Dr. Clark has developed her own parasite detection tester called a Syncrometer and a treatment machine called a Zapper. The latter is used as part of her treatment protocol that includes diet and various herbal products. The full details are included in her two books, "The Cure For All Cancers" and "The Cure For All Advanced Cancers". Her theories include the concept that parasites them-selves may have ingested viruses and fungi, so that any treatment that kills the parasite may thereby release into the body these other two infective agents. Her theories have led to conflict with the authorities, which should suggest that this treatment works and is therefore a threat to the drug orientated establishment. I have found that late onset diabetes can be the indirect result of a parasitic infection of the small bowel. In some cases of late onset diabetes the pancreas, as in acute onset diabetes, is damaged either by a parasite or a virus. However in many more instances the pancreas cannot produce insulin because of the deficiency of one or more of the three essential minerals chromium, vanadium and germanium.

Most patients can identify themselves with one or more of the above diseases. However this list is not exhaustive because anything that prevents the absorption of minerals can cause any of the symptoms and diseases associated with that particular deficiency or deficiencies. It is important to remember that many parasites excrete alcohol that can be absorbed through the gut wall. This means that patients may have all the same symptoms as an alcoholic. There may be a morning hangover, or even nausea. I have had patients just complaining of a hangover when they don't drink alcohol. Other patients seem to develop an allergy or hypersensitivity to alcohol that restricts their ability to drink it. Many patients are accused by doctors of being persistent drinkers of alcohol because the results of their various blood and other tests are identical to the investigations carried out on known alcoholics. At least one patient has had a drink drive conviction and maintains that she only had one unit of alcohol. Because most homoeopathic liquid medicines [known as remedies] contain large amounts of alcohol acting as a preservative, they are unsuitable for the treatment of alcohol producing parasites. If one of these remedies is used then the patient may experience severe side effects and then compelled to cease the treatment. Luckily we have discovered one American company that makes a limited number of remedies that contain no alcohol. Their range of alcohol free liquids includes two separate remedies that appear to treat most, if not all, alcohol-excreting parasites. Homoeopathic tablets designed to treat a specific parasite do not contain alcohol and therefore pose no problems associated with alcohol. However there are also several herbal remedies including black walnut and wormwood that are effective in treating parasites. The well-known herbal mixture known as essiac is also effective against some parasites, and this may explain its success in the treatment of some cancers.

Once the patient has recovered from the shock of being told that there is a parasite in their body, three questions follow. "How did I get them, can I pass them on to anyone else and how do I get rid of them?" I cynically say that the mere fact of living poses the threat of acquiring a parasite. Although the diagnosis of a parasite is rarely made by conventional medicine, American parasitologists have gone on record to claim that at least one in four people host a parasite at any one time, rising to one in two during their lifetime. They believe that modern lifestyles contribute to the problem, with the rapid movement by aeroplane, of both people and foods to and from those parts of the world where parasitic infections are endemic. More recent estimates suggest that the level of infestation has now risen to three out four people. This may sound bizarre but it does correlate with the rapid increase in all of the above diseases. Cancer is fast rising to affect one in every two people. Irritable bowel syndrome is estimated to affect one in five people and parasites are the commonest cause of this condition.

Parasites have a choice of three ways to enter the body. Namely through the mouth, lungs or skin. Obviously the commonest route into the body is via the mouth as a result of the contamination of food and drink. Both man and animals may contaminate any fruit and vegetable. The more primitive the working conditions for casual farm labourers, the more likely the accidental contamination of fruit and vegetables. Thus if any fruit or vegetable is eaten raw, it should be washed, preferably sterilised and possibly peeled. It is then difficult to gauge the balance between overcooking with the consequent destruction of nutrition, and undercooking which preserves the nutrition but runs the risk of failing to kill the parasites. Eating rare or undercooked meat could introduce a parasite into the body. Dirty hands or utensils may contaminate cold, but properly cooked meats. Smoked salmon can be harbouring a parasite, and therefore it is wise to freeze it before eating which should destroy any unwanted contaminants, prior to properly thawing it. Sushi, the rare fish delicacy, is a common source of parasites and it should carry a health warning that this raw fish is a common cause of parasitic infection. Even with the best of care it is impossible to identify the presence of various fish parasites before eating Sushi. It is therefore prudent to recommend that if Sushi is a favourite dish, to either have a test for parasites or have a regular course or anti-parasite treatment. Many people, especially in the USA, have a six monthly routine treatment to eradicate parasites. It is probably more sensible to do this rather than to rely upon the diagnosis of infestation, which can be very unreliable, unless the person conducting the investigation is very practiced in the detection of parasites.

Cold liquids can be contaminated. Even sophisticated water treatments can fail leading to contamination and, if this occurs and is recognised, water should be boiled before drinking. This contamination is usually noticed before too many people are exposed to infestation. However not all parasites are susceptible to routine water treatment. There is always the risk of contamination somewhere along the route between the water treatment works and the tap at the end of the supply chain. If the supply systems are damaged underground then unsuspected contamination can occur. Many people now use household water filters because of the common concern that water purification treatments are designed to remove infective agents, but not other pollutants. Other pollutants, like fluoride, may even be added at the treatment works. To remove fluoride is more difficult and may require a reverse osmosis filter system. I have found that in those patients who get frequent parasitic infections, a significant number do so due to drinking contaminated filtered water. I have now discovered that in some other countries its occurrence is well recognised and therefore documented that domestic filtered water is a possible source of infestation. Other cold liquids can pose a threat. It is possible to contaminate a liquid at source before it is sealed into its container. Liquids like milk can be contaminated, not only at source, but also during any part of the process of preparing cool dishes or drinks. Despite all the care that may be taken in the kitchen it is possible to contaminate food and drink either by careless handling or by some animal or insect. Some people adopt the extreme view that only food prepared in their own home is safe to eat. As a consequence of this view, as mentioned above, these people will take a course of anti-parasite treatment at least twice a year. If a food handler contaminates food with a bacteria or toxin then the victim is usually aware of the problem and soon develops diarrhoea and vomiting. However a person being infected by a parasite will most likely remain symptom free in the immediate period following that contaminated meal. However if there is a stomach upset following a parasitic contaminated meal then any symptoms are usually self limiting and soon forgotten, although at a later date there can be vague, and undiagnosed, abdominal symptoms.

It is possible for a parasite to enter the body through the skin. Walking barefooted on the grass or sand can expose the body to infestation. Other parasites can enter the body following a bite by an infected insect. Malaria is one example of an illness caused by a parasite entering through the skin as a result of a mosquito bite. There are several good books and audiotapes on the subject. A simple, and amusing guide to this subject can be found in "Guess what came to dinner" by Ann Louise Gittleman. Another book that offers simple advice is "The Parasite Menace" by Skye Weintraub.

Close bodily contact with an infected individual or animal is another source of infection. Threadworms in children lay their eggs around the anus. This causes irritation that in turn leads to scratching. If the fingers are then placed in the mouth in an act of comfort sucking, then the child re-infects itself. The eggs may also be thrown into the air when shaking the bedclothes and the eggs can then enter the body via the lungs and so produce a cough. In General Practice the only commonly recognised infection is by threadworms and it is not unusual to treat the whole family if a single member of the family is infected. However despite this common parasitic infection and the well-documented possible symptoms that it can cause (itching, waking with nightmares or vague abdominal pain), it is amazing how often there is a failure to make even this diagnosis.

The answer to the second question, "can I infect other people?" can now be answered by describing another source of infection. Possible infection between adults proves more difficult to cope with. Kissing, holding hands, and handling the same objects can lead to the transfer of parasites between adults. It is therefore not surprising that married couples or partners are prone to sharing each other's parasites. The more sexually active a couple then the more likely they will both be infected. This causes problems for the practitioner. It is uncommon to have both partners present for testing at the same time. Therefore you may successfully treat a patient, and in a short time they will reappear with another infestation. Since the partner may need a different treatment it is no good sending the patient home with a duplicate remedy for the partner to use. Further difficulties arise when the partner appears to be fully fit and cannot appreciate the necessity to be tested and treated. There may also be an element of guilt if the partner believes that he or she could be responsible for causing the ill health of the patient. Whenever the partner or other members of the family are present during the consultation I try to find time to carry out a quick test. It only takes one or two minutes to exclude parasites. Obviously if they are unwell it will take more time and therefore it is then necessary to make a further appointment.

So how do I get rid of parasites? It is possible to get rid of them by both conventional and alternative treatments. Conventional medicines are rarely used because of the frequent failure to detect the presence of parasites. Many doctors have yet to make the connection between diseases such as cancer diabetes and arthritis with the presence of parasites, and therefore it doesn't occur to them to look for these organisms. The main homoeopathic and herbal treatments that I use have been listed elsewhere. However for those patients who cannot obtain resonance homeopathic remedies, or if no suitable homoeopathic preparation can be found, there are other options available. Herbal products have been used for many hundreds of years for the treatment for parasites. There are various herbs available and I find that a mixture of black walnut and wormwood, available in capsule form, is both cheap and effective. If herbal tinctures are used instead of capsules, they carry the same potential side effects as described above because of their alcohol content. The capsular form of black walnut and wormwood is an ideal travel companion for those people who frequently have to journey to areas where there is a greater risk of infestation.

An herbal mixture known as essiac has worldwide reputation as a treatment for cancer. It is claimed that an elderly female patient told her Canadian nurse called Caisse (the letters of her name subsequently change to spell essiac) that a native Indian mixture containing four herbs had cured her breast cancer. This patient passed on to the nurse the recipe for this tribal treatment. The nurse eventually tried this herbal treatment on several terminally ill cancer patients, and had remarkably good results. This led to patients from all over North America seeking her help. Her results were confirmed by several doctors, but pressure from the medical authorities led to validation being withheld. Perhaps this is the first example of successful non-drug therapy being suppressed by the powerful medical and drug establishments. It must be understood that this tribal remedy is possibly hundreds of years old, and in Nurse Caisse's day cancer was a rare occurrence. In a previous chapter I have written about the six causes of all diseases. It seems very unlikely that the Indians suffered from viral and fungal illnesses. They were not immunised, had few if any modern environmental pollutants, and any possible genetic problems solved by a process of natural selection. This appears to leave only parasitic infection, perhaps understandable in view of their life style, as the most likely cause of illness. It is probable that the first elderly patient had a parasitic infestation, and hence the effect of essiac upon her parasites led to her recovery. It is likely that today's successes with essiac can be attributed to its anti-parasitic properties. Many people now take essiac as a preventive measure to diminish the probability that would develop cancer in the future. This is possibly equally effective as the more orthodox treatments for the prevention of parasitic diseases. Essiac is now available from a variety of sources, some containing just the original four herbal ingredients, although more correctly nurse Caisse added four more herbal ingredients during her work with the remedy.

Although I recommend people travelling to undesirable destinations that they should take with them one of these herbal capsules, there is however no substitute for general health precautions. These include avoiding the local water and ice. There are however sterilising products available, many however being chlorine based, to treat the water not only for drinking but also to soak, and so sterilise fruit and other uncooked foods. A dental mouthwash, called eliminator, made by Neways can safely be used to sterilise produce. It is also worthwhile avoiding cold foods like salad. Mention has been made of Dr Hulda Clark's Zapper device. This is another example of energy being used for treatment of parasites and also fungal and viral infections. I have described how resonance homoeopathic remedies work by destroying pathogens because of their susceptibility to specific harmonic vibrations. There is anecdotal evidence that the Zapper machine is effective in all three types of infection. The Zapper should be used at the end of the day when no further food and drink is to be taken and before retiring to bed. It is driven by a battery and has two electrodes, one for each hand. It is operated for three seven-minute periods separated by twenty-minute gaps. Dr Clark believes that the first treatment destroys the parasite, but that in death it releases any viruses or fungi that it may have devoured. The second and third treatments are designed to kill these other two pathogens.

One experimenter has studied the effects of a modified, and very portable machine the size of a cigarette packet, on various members of his family and reports great success in a variety of infections and has found that the age of the patient appears to be no barrier to safe effective treatment. If such a small device could be marketed it would be very useful in self-treatment, especially for those people with no knowledge of homoeopathy or herbal medicine, and who are deprived of access to orthodox medical treatment for parasites. This device being small and battery driven would be ideal to take away on any holiday or business trip. I have had experience of using both the original and the newer prototype and have found both to effective. A recent report on the use of a Zapper on tissue culture of cancer cells suggests that this machine is capable of causing a regression in their growth.

The real tragedy is that orthodox medicine possesses a good range of anti-parasitic medicines that are extremely effective.

Regrettably doctors choose to believe, or are taught, that parasites are very rare and therefore condemn many patients to years of misery and ill health. On a few occasions my patients have been bold enough to tell their G.P. or consultant that I have diagnosed the presence of parasites. This is usually dismissed as implausible but on more than one occasion the doctor has prescribed orthodox medical treatment just to prove that I was wrong. Invariably the patients recover, and a recent patient made a follow-up appointment specifically to tell the consultant that she hadn't been so well in years. A medical consultant who had spent time working in Africa did admit to me that if parasites were not suspected and specifically looked for, then it was most unlikely that they would be diagnosed even in hospital practice. If, as seems likely, a significant proportion of today's chronic illness is caused by parasites, then the failure of modern medicine to diagnose and treat them is directly responsible not only for overwhelming the NHS but also condemning countless patients to long term suffering. Is the doctor, or the system to blame?

The moral is that every one should be aware that parasite infections are very common and that any chronic illness should be considered to be due to the presence of a parasite until proved otherwise. Every attempt must be made to build up the body's immunity and to avoid any prescription or non-prescription medicine that has an antacid effect because the stomach's acid is part of the body's defence mechanism. Moreover any chronic dyspepsia is likely to be caused by a parasite. Take the preventative advice described above and avoid the trap of believing that you can do what you like and that modern medicine will cure all the consequences. Hospital wards and cemeteries are full of people who have made that mistake. Only one person can have your best interests at heart and that is **you**.

Chapter 19

Viral Illness: Doctors' Favourite Diagnosis

1960 to 1990 were the years of the virus. Despite the non-appearance of the anti-viral drug in chapter 3 all seemed under control. Epidemics came and went without great concern. As stated previously I have worked through 3 measles epidemics without experiencing any undue problems for the patients involved. The first 2 epidemics were spent in an urban practice with a generally young population. The number of house calls was very heavy on the alternate Mondays during the epidemic but the dire consequences attributed to measles by the pro-vaccination lobby failed to materialise.

However, these warnings have had an unsettling effect upon the present generation of doctors who have come to fear an epidemic of measles, polio and other potentially serious diseases. These doctors haven't seen the disease first hand, and I have seen several children who have been wrongly diagnosed as having measles. In retrospect, it is possible to assume that an antiviral drug would have reduced the level of immunity within the population, but would have caused far less long-term damage than appears to be the result of the ever-increasing vaccination programme.

Life for a GP was relatively simple. You soon learnt to identify the childhood viral illnesses. The only difficulty was an occasional mild form of mumps that failed to produce the very swollen face that stares out at you from the pages of medical textbooks. This left only the two remaining common viral illnesses, namely colds and influenza. In the earlier years of these three decades, influenza itself was relatively simple in that there appeared to be only two types, the 24 and 48-hour varieties. The employer would ask questions if anyone had a three-day absence attributed to influenza.

Then things started to go wrong. New viral illnesses started to be a problem. Glandular fever was one of the first new generation of diseases to appear in the Practice where I started my

144

medical career. Clinically it is difficult to diagnose because it presents itself in a variety of different forms. The initial diagnostic blood tests were unreliable. It was first reported in a London hospital where there was an epidemic amongst the nurses, medical students and young house doctors. Despite the fact that these young people had high temperatures and were off work, it was initially labelled as hysteria. Then it was named after the hospital concerned and even called the kissing disease. The latter description probably arose because of the habit of pathology departments to use throat swab cultures to determine which nurses were going out with which students or doctors. The use of the term 'kissing disease' has had an unfortunate consequence for many ill patients even today, more than 40 years since the disease was first recognised. It became accepted that it must be a disease confined to the late teens and early twenties. However age now appears to be no barrier and I regularly see this illness in both very young children and in the very elderly. The disease still presents itself in a variety of different forms, and is still very difficult, but not impossible, to diagnose from a purely clinical examination. With time restraints, and the inherent difficulty in making the diagnosis from a clinical examination, doctors generally opt for a diagnostic blood test. These blood tests are still not 100 per cent reliable, and because doctors have been taught that this is a disease of young adults, many patients outside this age group are even refused diagnostic blood tests. Consequently many patients remain undiagnosed, are often ill without due explanation, and many proceed to develop long-term chronic ill health. Glandular fever is therefore widespread amongst the population and continues to spread because the affected patients are unaware that they could pass on this virus to other people. A recent newspaper article claimed that a very high proportion of the population had glandular fever and that the virus remained in the body throughout the patient's life.

Diseases such as glandular fever do not conform to the previously adopted wisdom that viral illnesses were of short duration and were then followed by a complete recovery and generally life long immunity to that particular disease. By the mid sixties I was beginning to see an increasing number of very ill people who refused to make a quick recovery. Many continued to remain unwell for months and even years. This caused conflict with both employers and education authorities. Luckily, I had suffered a similar illness when at University. Then I was unwell for 2 months, and thereafter continued to get recurrent short-term illnesses. Because of my own experiences I had some sympathy with these patients. Over the following years a variety of labels have been applied to these patients. These have included post-viral illness, post-viral fatigue, post-viral syndrome and ME. Forty years later, and despite the fact that within the last few years ME has been recognised as a definite disease, many doctors continue to believe that it is a psychological problem rather than an organic illness and continue to believe that these patients should receive a long term course of anti-depressant drugs. The problem is further compounded by a variety of other chronic diseases that have acquired different names, different support groups and different 'specialists' but which all tend to rely upon various psychiatric drugs. In defence of orthodox medicine there have been various attempts to determine a specific cause for these diseases to justify the belief that a specific virus should be the sole cause of a specific disease.

The reality we now know is very different. Certainly the virus generally responsible for glandular fever can cause ME but it can also cause other illnesses like fibromyalgia. Conversely other viruses, and even non-viral infections, can cause ME as well as other chronic illnesses. The solution lies in the way that viruses reproduce. Viruses, like other forms of parasites, need a host body in which to reproduce. The virus enters the host either via the alimentary tract or the airway. The virus then selects a cell, which may be in a specific organ of the body depending upon the particular virus concerned. Having chosen the cell to be invaded, part of the virus enters into it and attaches itself to the nucleus of that cell. It then uses the nuclear materiel to create many new viruses. The cell is then packed with new viruses, but because the nucleus has been destroyed the cell dies, breaks down and releases these new viruses into the blood stream. This is associated with the episodes of fever that are so typical of influenza.

What happens next generally depends upon the state of the

146

body's immune system. Either the immune system mobilises its defence system to kill these viruses, with or without life-long immunity, or the virus will overwhelm the patient, who subsequently dies. There is however a third scenario. This assumes that a stalemate occurs in which neither the body nor the virus wins. The viral particle gets stuck in the nucleus and that in turn leads to the formation of an abnormal cell.

Sometimes the above process will be repeated as both the cell and the virus try to gain the upper hand, with recurrent low-grade illness that is so common with chronic glandular fever. It is also possible that the patient can recover spontaneously, especially when the immune system is boosted, but it is important to avoid any simultaneous overexertion during the period of debility. Too many athletes have paid the price for overexertion when faced with acute or chronic infection. The alternative to recurrent relapses is a state of chronic ill health because of the continued presence of abnormal cells with viral particles stuck in the nucleus. Normally the body removes abnormal cells, but in this case it appears incapable of doing so. The viral theory of cancer assumes that these abnormal cells with their virally damaged nuclei will eventually multiply to form a cancer. However as cancer is only one of many chronic illnesses a more general explanation for all these conditions must be sought. Therefore it is postulated that the abnormality leads to the body's inability to absorb one or more minerals that in turn results in illness. The form that the resulting illness takes will depend upon which minerals are involved and which of the several possibilities happen as a result of the failure to absorb these essential nutrients. This accords with the theory that all chronic disease is the result of a deficiency of one or more minerals

In the seventies it was quite common for doctors to diagnose a viral infection. This was partly due to the fact that the incidence of bacterial illnesses had been reduced due to antibiotics and the improvements in hygiene and sanitation. Therefore it was logical to attribute any acute symptoms of disease to the presence of a virus. Although specific blood tests for viruses still included many of the childhood illnesses, they omitted many other and possibly newer viruses. Although patients would have liked a specific

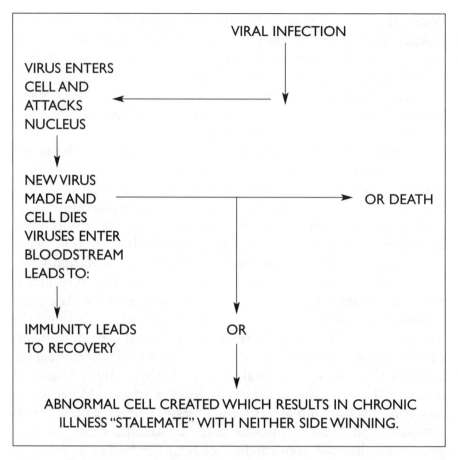

VIRAL INFECTION

VIRUS ENTERS
CELL AND
ATTACKS
NUCLEUS

NEW VIRUS
MADE AND   OR DEATH
CELL DIES
VIRUSES ENTER
BLOODSTREAM
LEADS TO:

IMMUNITY LEADS   OR
TO RECOVERY

ABNORMAL CELL CREATED WHICH RESULTS IN CHRONIC
ILLNESS "STALEMATE" WITH NEITHER SIDE WINNING.

name for their supposed viral illness, it was accepted that it was difficult to identify the specific organism. Therefore patients found reassurance in the diagnosis of a viral infection, and that their illness was genuine and 'not all in the mind'. This state of affairs existed until patients became more 'virus aware' and demanded more facts, coupled with the obvious fact that all types of illness were increasing and that the various health authorities were not coping with the upsurge in demand for medical care.

So why have all these changes taken place? We know that the effects of a virus can vary from patient to patient. It appears that a cold in one patient may reappear as influenza in another. Many mothers of large families will verify that if chicken pox affects their family it is usual to affect only one child at a time and that a severe case will be followed by a mild case before being followed by another severe case. I have already mentioned the different effects caused by a single virus in a family of four children totally isolated as a result of the snows of 1963.

It is further possible that with rapid travel by air new viruses can be introduced into communities that have no immunity to those particular viruses. This has happened before in history when native tribes had been decimated by the introduction of the measles virus to which they had no immunity. Some viruses, like the Ebola virus, have made the headlines, but other less virulent viruses may have escaped attention. Sometimes an epidemic of viral gastroenteritis that closes a hospital or a cruise ship will make the headlines. Some it is claimed, like the supposed AIDS virus appears to be a figment of imagination that has led to a very profitable source of income for the drug industry. So far there has been no published evidence that identifies one specific virus responsible for a set of symptoms known as AIDS. Computer generated images of a fictitious virus have been created and then accepted as a true magnified image of a real organism. Similarly the blood test used in the diagnosis of AIDS has been described as a scientific fraud and can produces positive results in a variety of other illnesses, and even false positives in healthy people. How is it possible to explain away the AIDS epidemic in Africa? These people continue to suffer a variety of other diseases, mainly parasitic and compounded by poor sanitation and inadequate nutrition. The drugs used to treat AIDS are themselves toxic and produce a wide variety of symptoms. Patients affected by AIDS when removed to places where there is better hygiene and also given a good diet appear to make a complete recovery. The sensible solution for Africa would appear to involve the transfer of money now spent upon drugs to enable improvements in sanitation, better quality drinking water and better nutrition. In my limited experience patients labelled as suffering from AIDS have parasitic infections leading to mineral deficiencies and the resulting consequences of those deficiencies.

Other viruses may be introduced via the immunisation programme. Certainly viruses have been altered before being introduced into vaccines. Some parents, who have not themselves been immunised against polio, have contracted poliomyelitis due to changing the nappy of a baby that had received a recent poliomyelitis vaccine. Finally a population whose health and immunity have been compromised by a variety of causes may be susceptible to hitherto non-pathogenic viruses. However for whatever reason acute and chronic viral infections have increased to epidemic proportions and that this has been accompanied by an increase in all chronic diseases that may even require hospital admission.

The recent SARS virus epidemic is a prime example of how the media can be involved in a hysterical and unreasonable response. Despite the fact the source of this virus, its mode of origin and how it was spread were all unknown, an extraordinary chain reaction occurred that frightened people and caused financial problems for many countries and their various industries.

Was the SARS virus the result of various animals being kept in cages and in close proximity to one another? Recent articles suggest that the epidemic started in parts of China where cats, bred for human consumption, were kept caged in close proximity to one another. It can of course happen again. It is known that animals kept in poor conditions are prone to disease and that such diseases can spread to humans. If the human beings themselves have poor immunity they too can develop severe symptoms. Was it further spread because of a poor or damaged sewage system? One newspaper article claimed that it could be caught from a door handle previously touched be an infected person. Had the virus been accidentally or deliberately released into the environment following a scientific experiment or even during the manufacture of a vaccine? Whatever the reasons we were shown pictures of people wearing masks and spraying everything with various solutions, even though both exercises may have been worthless. Were we supposed to demand the production of a vaccine for worldwide immunisation against this disease? It is sobering to remind ourselves that many more people have died as a result of influenza, famine, war or other similar disasters.

So how do we treat viral infections? There are basically two types of infection, acute and chronic. Most of us suffer from a variety of acute viral illnesses; the problems occurring when the body is unable to rid itself of the virus and consequently descends

150

into a sate of chronic ill health. I use resonance homoeopathic remedies to treat both acute and chronic viral illnesses. In chronic illness resonance homoeopathic remedies shake the viral particles away from the cell nucleus. The viral particles are then expelled from the cell and out into the blood circulation. The final, but important, part of treatment involves the consumption of copious amounts of water intended to sweep along the offending viral particles and so out of the body via the kidneys. It is assumed that if these viral particles are not promptly eliminated from the body they could be capable of recovering their energy. These revitalised viruses would then be capable of re-entering new cells and starting the same process over again. Glandular fever has been frequently mentioned in this chapter, so that it is worth mentioning that this and other chronic infections if treated in this manner can lead to a complete recovery, but unfortunately still leaving the patient without immunity to that particular virus. Therefore the treated patient should be warned that they are susceptible to further infection if they are exposed to the virus at some date in the future, and that it is wrong to assume that the same illness cannot recur.

I realise that the resonance theory is mentioned elsewhere in this book but it was in the context of chronic viral illness that Dr. Helmut Schimmel first introduced me to these remedies. Dr. Schimmel had spent many years developing both the remedies and machines that are today in widespread use, especially in Germany. He believed that viruses were responsible for the majority of cancers. Other German doctors have developed similar resonance remedies and similar diagnostic machines. The theories of resonance have been taken up by other companies and are now widely used in the treatment, not only of infective organisms, but also to restore the vitality of different organs of the body. Although there has been a concerted campaign to denigrate homoeopathy, there are thousands of people who can testify that resonance remedies have safely and effectively cured conditions that drug-based medicines have failed to relieve. In this respect the logic of physics has triumphed over the profit driven trial and error of the pharmaceutical chemistry. NASA too has been involved in the research and development of bio energy concepts.

(Since writing this chapter I have learnt of the sad death of Dr Schimmel).

It may seem slightly odd to have started with the chronic diseases before the acute ones. However this was a deliberate decision because chronic viral infections are notoriously difficult to treat and resonance homoeopathy remains my gold standard for their treatment. However there are a great variety of other products that can be used to treat acute viral infections and also to prevent or minimise the effects of such diseases. The treatment of chronic viral illness doesn't cease with the above therapy. If nothing else was done the patient would be left free of the virus but in a debilitated state and easy prey for any other infective agent that happened to come along. It is essential to rebuild the patient's immunity and vitality. There will be mineral deficiency either as a result of the infection or was the pre-existing reason why the patient was susceptible to the infection. Therefore supplementation with the previously recommended mineral solutions should be commenced at an early stage. The use of these minerals solutions is but one example of how a product can be used in both the treatment and prevention of an illness. A good antioxidant mixture is also essential not only in the treatment but in the prevention of other infections. Cordyceps mushroom extract that is present in a Neways' herbal mixture called Ming Gold that is used to boost physical performance, appears to have some antiviral properties and some people will use this product at the first sign of developing a cold or influenza. If a patient is denied access to a resonance remedy it is worth trying this herbal product together with an antioxidant, both in high doses and in combination with mineral solutions. A zapper may also be of benefit. When I treat cancer, or a similar serious illness, I always treat the underlying condition first. If the underlying cause is found to be a virus then I would treat it in the above manner, before any consideration is given to the addition of the other cancer fighting products. This is also the time to consider treatments like B17, Vitamin C and Essiac. Mangosteen has anti-viral, anti-fungal, anti-bacterial and anti-parasitic actions.

There are many different products available to treat or alleviate acute viral infections. There is a range of resonance remedies to suit different viruses, even one specifically designed to treat the glandular fever virus. For those people sensitive to alcohol there is an alcohol free remedy made in the USA.. In addition there are a variety of flower essence based remedies, mainly originating from the Pacific region. The Himalayan region also produces a remarkably effective product that is both antiviral and antibiotic. Increased doses of antioxidants have been shown to alleviate the effects of viral infection. Red wine has been shown to contain antioxidants glycoproteins and anti-fungal agents. A recent report claims that two daily glasses of red wine reduces the chances of developing a cold by 50per cent. Several other products have been demonstrated to have some antiviral activity. The same is true of Noni juice a polysaccharide product of the Pacific and Caribbean regions that has been used by those native cultures for many different illnesses. Various aromatherapy products, including lavender and frankincense, have antiviral properties and can either be used to protect the individual, or to limit the spread of airborne viruses in a public area. Lavender oil rubbed into the nose is claimed to protect against cold and flu when in a crowded bus, train, ship or aeroplane, especially when there is re-circulation of the air.

Prevention of acute illness should be the main aim of any therapy. If that fails then every attempt is made to reduce its severity and prevent the progression to chronic illness. I believe that liquid mineral solutions and antioxidant supplementation on a daily basis are both essential. Different approaches have been tried and most people have their own favourite products. The various options may also include separate vitamin C supplementation. Many years ago it was shown that zinc reduced cold symptoms, and many people take extra zinc at the first signs of a cold. Substances that enhance the body's immune system should be encouraged, and many of these contain echinacea. Mention of lavender and frankincense in protection when exposed to a possible threat has already been mentioned. Chapter 21 deals with the problems of immunisation, but at this point I would urge caution in relying upon annual influenza immunisation. Firstly it doesn't replace the need for supplementation and immune system boosters. Secondly a significant number of people remain unwell following the administration of the vaccine. If any immunisation is desired it is safer to rely upon the homoeopathic cold and flu remedy, the ingredients of which vary on an annual basis in a similar fashion to the conventional vaccine injection. Neither of these methods is of use if an unexpected strain of virus appears in the community. There are also some flower essence vaccines and also a Photobiophysics vaccine.

Despite having covered only two of the six major causes of disease, it is possible to appreciate how parasites and viruses have been responsible for so much human misery, ill health and death. Equally obvious is the fact that the world would be very different if these two pathogens had been treated by the various methods so far described. However it is the marked contrast in approach to the two diseases that causes most concern. Medical practice is very closely regulated and therefore it is safe to assume that the manner in which doctors treat disease receives the tacit approval and support of both government and the drug industry.

Worldwide parasites are probably the commonest pathological cause of illness. Doctors have at their disposal an embarrassingly large array of medicines capable of killing parasites. It would seem logical to use these treatments to heal people and at the same time enhance the medical profession's reputation. The reverse is true and doctors steadfastly refuse to accept the concept of parasitic illness. This conflicts with the Hippocratic concept of medical practice. It is worth repeating that this state of affairs cannot persist without the tacit approval of government, and the connivance of the drug companies.

The very reverse situation occurs with viruses. Doctors are more than happy to make the diagnosis of a viral infection, even in the absence of this pathogen. Presumably their attitude is inspired by the knowledge that there is no known anti viral drug that would prove or disprove the accuracy of their diagnosis. Thus ill health prevails and we are left with the inescapable conclusion that the various authorities are content with the present high levels of illness. The totally different medical approach to these two major causes of illness defies all logic.

There is another, and moral, aspect to the medical approach that involves AIDS and the disastrous effects that this disease is having in the African continent. We are constantly told that that Aids poses a major threat to Africa and that the various governments are ensuring that various "cut price" drugs are being made available to treat it. These drugs are not cures and they have considerable toxic side effects that are indistinguishable from some of the symptoms ascribed to the disease itself. Many of these drugs are not licensed as safe in the western world. We have therefore suffered forty years of avoidable illness since the withdrawal of anti viral wonder drug in 1962. These same forty years have yielded ongoing revenue for the drug companies in respect of vaccines and other drugs. AIDS has therefore been allowed to become a license for drug companies to continue to profit from illness. It could of course eventually become the Achilles heel of both companies and governments.

If AIDS is indeed a viral illness then either the original drug or a modern equivalent, or even resonance homoeopathy, could, or should, have been used to rid the African continent of this disease. Again if it is not the result of a virus then Africa has been the victim of a gigantic international fraud. If it is not a viral illness, then the vast sums of money spent on drugs would have been better employed providing anti parasitic drugs, clean water and good nutrition. Presumably there is little desire, on the part of certain political organisations, to see Africa populated by large numbers of healthy people.

Chapter 20

Fungal Infections: The Candida Theories

Everyone has heard of candida. Fungal infections are common and most difficult to successfully treat. Dermatologists have to cope with both skin and nail infections. The latter is notoriously difficult to treat and it takes many months treatment before being rewarded by healthy looking nails. Most women have experienced vaginal thrush (candida). For the majority of women one course of treatment usually cures the condition and it never recurs. Other women are less fortunate and their lives are blighted by frequent relapses. Worse still, thrush may be mistaken for a urinary infection leading to a course of antibiotics and a consequent worsening of the thrush. Other women are labelled as having recurrent urinary infections, and are treated accordingly with long-term antibiotics. Eventually the long-term sufferer may be referred to a consultant gynaecologist, who also wrestles with the problem, but again treatment is often unsuccessful. These poor unfortunate women are then written off as inevitably chronic patients with devastating consequences not only for their sex lives, but also for their general mental and physical well being. Frequently a parasitic infection can mimic both thrush and urinary infection, but when the parasite is treated the symptoms attributed to the other illnesses will disappear.

However fungal infections are not confined to the skin, nails and vagina. Many patients, mostly women, also suffer with fungal infections of the bowel, and less commonly in other regions of the body including the brain. Regrettably these unfortunate people have difficulty in persuading doctors that such infections do exist. The exception to this general rule is where a patient's immune system is so compromised as a result of medical treatment that there is a rapid spread of some fungal infection throughout the body. Examples of this medically induced condition are found in those patients who are receiving long term high doses of steroids, or who are receiving treatment for the so called AIDS virus. Those patients who have been cast aside by mainstream medicine either have to suffer in silence or resort to seeking advice and help from the various self-help groups, or from an alternative health practitioner

Throughout the rest of this chapter I will use the term candida instead of fungus because it is a word universally recognised possibly because it is regarded as the commonest form of all such infections. Why has it become such a problem? It is a naturally occurring organism, present in most, if not all, people and normally lives in harmony with all the other organisms that inhabit our bodies. It only comes to our notice when it multiples in number and replacing other organisms and so creating the symptoms that the patient can no longer ignore. There are several possible reasons why this can happen. Decades of antibiotic misuse (including the antibiotics in food) and the introduction of the oral contraceptive pill in the early sixties have both been blamed. Stomach acid is designed to kill candida in food and therefore any of the modern medicines introduced to neutralise or prevent acid formation may cause problems. Modern antibiotics are stronger and are capable of killing more and more organisms leaving the field clear for the growth of candida that is resistant to these medicines. Bubble baths, fabric softeners and stockings being replaced by tights have all received the finger of suspicion. Chronic sufferers of vaginal candidiasis are advised to avoid the last three possible culprits. Food and drinks with high sugar content, and alcohol, certainly aggravate candida present in the bowel and may even be the original cause of the condition. So many things in our environment have changed that is difficult to avoid food contaminated by antibiotics, cortisones and hormones. Sugars and refined carbohydrates are difficult to avoid due to their presence in so many items of food and drink. You only have to read the diet sheets recommended by the various support groups to realise how difficult it is to avoid all these ingredients. So many of the chemicals in use today that can be present in toiletries, personal care products or perfumes may either enhance the growth of candida directly or by inhibiting the growth of competing organisms. Perhaps the most potent reason for the increase in this condition has been the decline in the general levels of immunity. Candida and other fungal infections are often a feature in patients with chronic viral and parasitic infections. It is a rule of thumb that viral infections should be treated as a first priority, and quite often the candida will cease to be a problem once the virus has been eliminated and immunity restored by the use of minerals, vitamins and antioxidants. In my opinion the state of the immune system is the key, and once the six main possible ill-health factors have been removed, proper nutrition restored and environmental pollutants avoided, then the body's immune system will revert to its normal healthy level to do the job it was designed to do. Candida, a common feature in cancer patients, is probably the result of lowered immunity, either as part of the original disease process or as a result of conventional cancer therapy, rather than the cause of the cancer itself.

Candida infection of the bowel causes a variety of symptoms that can be loosely classified as irritable bowel syndrome (IBS). When parasitic infection has been excluded candida is the most likely cause of IBS. The sufferers are predominately female and the symptoms rarely begin before the later teenage years. The exceptional appearance at a younger age is often due to parasites acquired from a family pet or long term antibiotic use for chronic infections or acne. At this age the introduction of oral contraceptives, tights and the increase use of various personal care products to enhance beauty can easily be associated with, and blamed for, the onset of abdominal symptoms. There can be pain, distension, wind in both directions and alteration in the bowel habits. Rarely alcohol can be produced in the bowel and lead to symptoms associated with an excess alcohol intake. Alcohol feeds cancer cells and therefore may also be the original cause of the cancer. The symptoms may be similar to those produced by alcohol excreting parasites, however in the case of parasites there are usually less in the way of abdominal symptoms. This is possibly due to the different methods of generating alcohol. In parasites the alcohol is formed within the parasite and then excreted as a waste product. In candida it appears to be formed by a process of fermentation leading to 'frothing' and distension of the bowel. Abdominal distension has become so common as a symptom that it is often dismissed by doctors as being an unfortunate consequence of being a woman. Many women come to accept this state of affairs, but they begin to worry about possible cancer after reading in the newspapers about other women developing ovarian cysts or cancer that had grown to the size of a football before being distinguished from simple distension. The uncertainty can result in repeated visits to the doctor seeking reassurance, but unfortunately leading to being labelled as a neurotic patient. This can often be resolved by lying flat on the back when a distended abdomen will slowly subside and remain soft to the touch. If a cyst, cancer or even a large uterus is present then, on lying down, there will be less lowering of the abdominal wall and the swelling will feel firm or even hard. To have both conditions can be both confusing and unlucky. However for these women a routine self-examination is as useful as self-examination of their breasts. In turn it will result in fewer wasted visits to the doctors.

In time the patient will discover various factors that appear to affect the severity of symptoms. Certain foods seem to rapidly lead to symptoms, and these invariable include sugars and refined starch. The patient will come to notice an apparent allergy to an increasing number of different foods. Food and drink containing yeast and sugars will often set off a reaction. Bread and cakes will soon be added to the list of foods to be avoided. This may or may not lead to wheat sensitivity, and a wheat free diet is not easy to follow. Although help may be refused via the health system it is now possible to obtain wheat and yeast free products. The patient may find that certain alcohol products, like wine and beer, soon lead to problems whereas some spirits may not. It will depend upon the method of alcohol production and whether fermentation has taken place.

Patients may seek advice from the various self-help groups. These organisations will offer dietary advice. The diets are not easily followed, but such is the desperation of these patients that they will adhere to the diet to be rid of their distressing symptoms. They will find that any indiscretion will lead to a violent reaction. This is due to the nature of candida and other fungi. Without their food they will convert into a seed or spore form. They will remain inert within the body until their required food reappears. It is like the desert flowers whose seeds lie dormant in the sand for many years, but within hours of a rainstorm the desert will bloom with flowers. It is therefore obvious that a diet is not a long-term solution. Neither does it solve the problem of allergies that have developed during the period of candidiasis, even though the food items themselves may not be essential for the metabolism of candida. It is therefore obvious that diet alone is not a solution but a cure must be found. Dietary advice alone is not in the long term interest of patients and can even lead to a worsening of health.

The allergies that occur during the course of this infection are attributed to the presence of a 'leaky gut'. It is assumed that the filaments of the candida bore their way in the walls of the intestine like a corkscrew into the cork of a bottle. This leaves a hole on the wall of the intestine that allows undigested food to enter the body. Because this food form is alien to the body (i.e. not broken down into the component parts that should be normally absorbed) its immune system comes into play and an allergic reaction is created that will reappear every time the patient eats that particular food.

However that is not the whole story. In accordance with my basic rule, which states that with any illness there is always a mineral deficiency that is resistant to supplementation until the infection or other cause is treated first. With any allergy there is invariably a deficiency of zinc. There may be other deficiencies too that will account for the other symptoms that coexist with the bowel problem. There may be tiredness, ME or any other chronic illness. However because routine estimation of mineral content is not part of medical practice it is impossible to say if a resistant mineral deficiency is the cause or the result of the candida infection. Therefore with an ill patient we are always left with the need to treat the infection and then introduce minerals into the body.

Treatment of candida and other fungal infections is far from easy. Some patients have to continue for a long period of time taking a maintenance dose of a herbal combination. Homoeopathic medicines are unsuitable for long-term use. However I believe that treatment is often unsuccessful because of some other underlying condition which itself may not be apparent. The patient may keep suffering repeated re-infection from a partner, in much the same manner as parasites may be reintroduced before treatment is satisfactorily completed. In the first few days of treatment the patient may experience extra symptoms due to the dead and dying candida before these organisms are expelled from the body. The patient must be warned about a variety of possible unpleasant reactions, which may seem worse than the original illness, and should be encouraged to persevere with treatment despite the temptation to stop it. These side effects usually last a few days and can be minimised by drinking copious volumes of water.

I do not believe that a rigid diet is necessary because the spores are more difficult to treat than the living organism. However some conventional medical treatments fail because sugar is added to the medicine itself to make it more palatable. This is particularly true of the oral thrush of babies who become infected either at birth or from the teat of a feeding bottle. There are sugar free treatments available, but their existence is not readily brought to the attention of doctors. It is sometimes necessary to use this sugar free baby formula on adults, but obviously in higher doses than for infants. As with viral and parasitic infections there are several effective resonance homoeopathic remedies for the treatment of candida and other fungal infections. The remedies are particularly useful when candida affects the brain because of the difficulty in getting treatments to the brain itself. These patients with cerebral candida describe how, with a flare-up of infection, there is a sudden onset of tiredness, as if a curtain descends that shuts down the brain functions. In early infections simple homoeopathic candida 30C may be effective. Of the herbal remedies those combinations containing caprilic acid are generally the most effective. Essiac also has anti-fungal activity. A course of treatment using a Zapper is worthwhile. For nail infections origano aromatherapy oil rubbed into the base of the nail may be effective. There are several flower essences that have anti-fungal properties. Xango (mangosteen) juice has potent anti-fungal activity and is very effective in fungal nail infections.

In conclusion fungal infection can be very resistant to

treatment. They often coexist with, or are the result of, other pathological conditions. However when these other problems are dealt with candida suddenly becomes amenable to treatment, even vanishing spontaneously. This is one condition that should be avoided, and lifestyle choices adopted that will make the body a hostile environment for candida and other fungi. Although candida infections are more commonly associated with women, men too suffer from this.

Chapter 21

Immunisation: Every Parent's Dilemma

There is no doubt in my mind that any vaccine is capable of damaging health. The important question is how and why they cause damage, and how can that damage be repaired? Although MMR vaccines dominate the media, other stories continue to reappear, including various problems associated with the two Gulf wars. We should be concerned about the number of newer vaccines that have been promised to treat or prevent a wide variety of diseases.

Immunisation is probably the most contentious issue in medicine and politics. Several major court cases are pending which claim vaccine damage due to the MMR vaccine. This is likely to be the first major issue on vaccines facing the English Courts. However there are other cases pending both in the UK and USA that involve other vaccines. Parents are increasingly concerned and worried about the possible side effects of vaccines. The Government continues to insist that vaccines are 100 per cent safe, despite the fact that specific vaccines or even batches of vaccines have had to be withdrawn when the number and magnitude of the side effects could not be ignored. This is also foolhardy because I know of nothing in medical practice that is 100 per cent safe. In Japan the MMR vaccine has been withdrawn because of unacceptable reactions. Government claims that this was a faulty type of vaccine, and only our brand of MMR is safe. Parents who believe that this triple vaccine is suspect find it is difficult to obtain the single vaccines. The excuse of manufacturers is that the triple vaccine is so popular that the demand for the single varieties has fallen and therefore their production is not commercially viable! Parents would be prepared to accept a high percentage of vaccine safety if, when things went wrong, it was immediately acknowledged and that help was available. In the meantime the vaccine uptakes are falling and every single episode of measles is treated like a national emergency. There is so much political and financial pressure behind vaccine programmes that a major confrontation with the public seems inevitable.

Despite the public concerns, the pharmaceutical industry and governments are pressing to produce and then introduce further new or combination vaccines. There seems to be a drive to create a vaccine for almost every medical condition except, it appears, for vaccine damage itself. Where damage is suggested, it will never be found because instead every effort will be made to discredit such claims. The proof of damage is easily found, but there continues to be determined efforts to prevent any research that is likely to implicate vaccines. In America attempts are being made to create a compulsory immunisation programme with children receiving vaccines before going to school. However even in America, the litigation against vaccine manufacturers had reached such a point that it threatened to bankrupt the whole immunisation programme. The American Government has stepped in to protect the manufacturers by meeting the claims for damages from tax revenues, but only acknowledges the most severe reactions that arise soon after the injection of the vaccine. This is but the tip of an iceberg because as explained later in this chapter the majority of the reactions are delayed and seem to bear no relation to the immunisation procedure itself. Governments have discouraged all long-term studies preferring to record only the short-term acute reactions.

I have no doubt whatsoever that any vaccine is capable of damaging health. Other countries quietly accept that damage occurs. In Germany, a country we laud for their good health care system, machines are manufactured that can detect vaccine damage. Parents know this and are aware that damage does occur, and that there are ways in which it can be treated. On the Continent there is not the same hysterical response from the various governments and the media.

The real problem arises because of medicine's obsession that for a vaccine to cause any damage it must cause the same condition every time. This is why statistical evidence fails to prove a link between two events, like MMR and autism. There is no doubt in my mind that the MMR vaccine can lead to autism, but it can also lead to other illnesses as well. Other vaccines can also

164

cause autism as well as other diseases. The other confusing problem for the statisticians is that it isn't possible to state that it is the measles component of the vaccine that causes the damage. For autism to occur there must always be a marked deficiency of selenium, which may even predate the vaccine injection or be caused by it. There is usually in addition a deficiency of lecithin or another essential fatty acid. Other deficiencies may coexist. Heredity will be examined in greater detail in the next chapter, but a child may be short of selenium purely because its mother was also deficient and didn't have enough to pass on to the child either via the umbilical cord or in breast milk. If the child itself cannot absorb selenium then it seems to be far more likely to suffer vaccine damage. Sometimes it is what is passed from mother to unborn infant that is important, rather than what is missing. I have found vaccine damage in unvaccinated infants, passed to them from mothers who themselves had unsuspected vaccine damage. Polio and tetanus vaccine damage seem to be the commonest form of disease passed from mother to infant. These two vaccines have been in use for many years and therefore in the future we may see more examples of damage caused by the newer vaccines like the MMR being passed from mother to child. Therefore it is feasible for even an unvaccinated child to develop autism, or indeed any other disease.

So how can vaccines cause damage? There are several theories, and any one or combination could feasibly cause it. In appendix E you will find a list of fillers that are used in the manufacture of vaccines. There are several of these fillers including mercury that are known to be neurotoxic chemicals (i.e. can damage nerve tissue). It is feasible to postulate that the large number of injections given in such a short space of time could add up to a total amount of mercury that exceeds the safe levels and that this fact alone could be responsible for autism and other diseases of the nervous system. In January 2003 there were press reports that, of the flu vaccines given in the autumn of 2002, 70 per cent contained mercury. As expected the Department of Health claimed that the vaccine was 100 per cent safe.

Then there is the so-called active ingredient of the vaccine. It is usually altered in some way so that it is supposed to impart immunity without causing the actual disease. This has certain problems not the least of which is the fact that it may not lead to immunity which is why even immunised people sometimes succumb to the disease that they are supposed to be protected from. Other people will develop an illness to the infective agent that was supposed to protect against the targeted disease. Is this a possible cause for some of the new strains of viral diseases that are appearing?

What is the prospect of an AIDS vaccine being manufactured and used to combat an AIDS virus that has not been demonstrated to even exist?

Some people will be ill for weeks or even months after receiving the influenza vaccine demonstrating that damage from immunisation is no respecter of age. It is also difficult to assess the level of immunity by blood estimation in health care professionals who need to be protected against Hepatitis B. This can lead to unnecessary re-immunisation in the hope that blood tests would suggest that the worker has achieved immunity to Hepatitis B. This is a concern because it questions the theory of immunity or even of past infection by the estimation of specific antibody levels to a specific disease. Some of these vaccines may have been manufactured with contact to yeast and thus could cause a reaction in yeast sensitive people. The theory of immunisation is possibly fatally flawed because there will be a decline in naturally acquired immunity resulting from infection to a specific disease. Some defence against the contents of the vaccine given will replace this naturally acquired immunity. Therefore in years to come there may be a re-emergence of major epidemics due to diseases that were in many cases already declining prior to the immunisation cult. This natural immunity has been replaced by at best possible immunity to man made diseases. If the theory of immunisation was discredited and stopped, there could be epidemics of the man-made diseases in addition to the original diseases. If you would like more information on the flawed theory of immunisation from the days of Edward Jenner (the originator of smallpox vaccination) and all the consequences of its implementation, I would suggest reading "The Sanctity of Blood, vaccination is not immunisation" by Tim O'Shea.

166

Another book that is equally damning is, "the Vaccination bible" by Lynne McTaggart.

Whatever the cause and method of vaccine damage, one essential fact remains. In all cases there is a deficiency of one or more minerals, possibly also associated with some vitamin and essential fatty acid deficiencies, but resistant to supplementation unless combined with additional treatment for the vaccine damage itself. In this respect diseases arising from vaccine damage do so in the identical manner to parasitic, viral and fungal infections. Similar disease mechanisms will be described in Chapters 22 and 23. In all these cases the presenting illness is the result of one or more of the diseases/symptoms attributed to the specific mineral deficiencies. Conversely mineral deficiency seems to leave patients more susceptible to damage from immunisation.

In my experience vaccine damage is responsible for the majority of chronic illness found in young children. Asthma, eczema and allergies are usually due to a zinc deficiency. Lack of zinc also reduces the immunity and the child could suffer frequent colds and this combined with dairy sensitivity leading to catarrh, glue ear, deafness and probably unnecessary operations. Recent research claims that excessive use of antibiotics before the age of 6 months results in an allergy before 7 years. Why should a healthy immune baby need antibiotics so early in life? In addition to rare genuine conditions there seems to three possible reasons. Firstly error in the need for antibiotics, and secondly a child born with a defective immune system as a result of the mother's illness. Thirdly vaccine damage, remembering that by 6 months a child will have already received a cocktail of vaccines.

The symptoms of allergies asthma and allergy will appear even when there is minimal zinc deficiency. Therefore it is not unusual to be told that a child has suffered eczema since birth, but mother has forgotten that the first immunisation was probably given at around 2 months of age. If it were due to simple poor nutrition then supplementation that includes zinc would lead to a rapid improvement in the child's skin. It may also need a fatty acid like primrose oil, but this simple deficiency is fairly rare, because it is often associated with other deficiencies. Hyperactivity in young children can be due to sensitivity to sugar and colourings, again due to a shortage of zinc. Selenium deficiency is also often found in hyperactivity and other behavioural and education problems. Hyperactivity is just one of the conditions that are causing problems within the education system. In December 2002 official government figures suggest that one in every twenty children aged between six and twenty years of age requires Ritalin or a similar drug to dampen severe hyperactivity that could lead to violence. If you are concerned about the effects of Ritalin then I would suggest that there is ample evidence readily available that this drug's adverse effects far outweigh any potential benefits. If in doubt read the makers of Ritalin's own published list of side effects. In England and America it is estimated that one in five children has special educational needs, ranging from this simple allergic hyperactivity to the more serious conditions like autism. Again the majority of these conditions have either an element of deficiency or far more likely the symptoms are totally due to it. If the child is born with a normal supply of selenium it appears to be less susceptible to suffer vaccine damage. However if there is vaccine damage and selenium is the only mineral involved there may be a total lack of symptoms for years or even decades. For some reason, unlike zinc the body appears to cope until the body's stores of selenium are almost totally depleted. However if for any reason the child is born with minimal or no selenium, there is not only a greater risk of vaccine damage, but any symptoms will appear earlier and with an increased possibility of developing one of the neurological or educational problems. Zinc and selenium deficiencies are by far the commonest found in young children, and the conditions mentioned here are also the most likely to occur. However, any deficiency and any medical problem can occur and should be excluded especially if they have severe implications for the family. Is epilepsy developed at an early age due to a congenital abnormality, the result of damage during birth or an infection of the brain? Before accepting one of these permanent conditions it is important to exclude vaccine damage and a deficiency that can be reversed. University students who have received meningitis vaccination can suddenly develop epilepsy. In general the early appearance of the conditions like eczema are due to the polio vaccine, whereas those conditions that appear later and involving selenium deficiency are generally due to tetanus vaccine or one of the ingredients of MMR. With every new vaccine or combination of vaccines there are greater future health risks for the recipients.

As already mentioned vaccine damage can occur at any age, but children are more susceptible because of the immaturity of their immune system and the large number of vaccines that they receive over a relatively short period of time. Damage in latter years depends upon circumstances. Entrants to the health care professions are required to have not only booster injections but also to receive a course of Hepatitis B vaccines. People who travel, or may travel, as a consequence of their employment also are required to have up to date vaccine cover. Members of the armed forces who fought in the Gulf War were given a cocktail of vaccines and other chemicals that has probably contributed to various conditions like the Gulf War Syndrome. Although the role of vaccination has been dismissed, the official investigators do not know how to test for vaccine damage; neither do they measure all the mineral levels in the body. In December 2002 the armed forces were preparing for a possible invasion of Iraq. At least one national paper reported that soldiers were refusing the voluntary anthrax vaccine because they didn't believe the Ministry of Defence claims that the vaccine was totally safe. New recent reports link multiple abortions, deaths and congenital abnormalities amongst the children of service personnel from certain units who had received the anthrax vaccine. Airline crews are similarly required to maintain up to date vaccinations so that they are free to fly anywhere in the world. Unlike most service personnel they are free to consult civilian doctors, and those doctors who see large numbers of aircrew, share my view that a significant number are suffering vaccine damage. All people who travel on holiday for pleasure may be advised to receive booster doses or may be required to possess proof of yellow fever vacci-nation. I have seen several cases of problems following yellow fever injection. Influenza vaccine can often cause problems, and you only have to stand in a Post Office queue to hear the comment that, "I haven't been well since I had my flu jab". Until there is routine estimation of the body's minerals patients will continue to suffer ill health and politicians and doctors will continue to proclaim that vaccination is safe. Both have a vested interest in the immunisation programme. In Britain every patient that is persuaded to have the influenza vaccine (or indeed any other recognised immunisation) earns the doctor a significant extra fee, and so patients are encouraged to queue for their injections, each and every year.

General practitioners receive from the Government extra income for various services that includes childhood immunisation. However doctors only receive this additional income when they have completed the required course of injections for a very high proportion of the children registered with their practice. If only a very few families refuse the immunisation of their children the doctors will receive **no** additional income despite immunising the majority of children. When faced with the prospect of a potential loss of income is it any wonder that doctors and their staff will exert undue influence upon parents to persuade them to comply with the immunisation protocol? It is easy to appreciate how possible it could be to discard honesty, integrity and any acceptance of the possibility of vaccine damage when so much is at stake. Although the system of additional payments was introduced with the best of motives, the increasing concerns over vaccine safety has turned an incentive into an inducement.

So what are the alternatives? Firstly, to understand the reason for a given immunisation and, secondly, to ensure that you are fully fit to receive the vaccine and that there is no mineral deficiency. It is a requirement not to inject if the patient has, or appears to have, an infection on the day of the appointment. However the pressures, both financial and political, may encourage the doctor or nurse to ignore this advice due to pressure of work, or because a baby has missed too many previous appointments due to ill health. There are homoeopathic versions of all the commercial vaccines and can be used either to immunise, or to reverse the damage caused by a specific vaccine, or in some cases administered at the same time as the injection to minimise side effects. This is a classical homoeopathic approach that had been used for many years to desensitise people before desensitising vaccines were produced. These remedies are once again being

170

used because of the potential possible harmful effects of desensitising vaccines that can even rarely include death of the patient. We regularly use homoeopathic vaccines to successfully treat vaccine damage. An increasing number of patients choose to use homoeopathic vaccines in lieu of the orthodox injections. This is particularly true of people who choose the homoeopathic cold and flu vaccine rather than the injection. It appears to be very effective and is made from the same strains of virus as used in the injected vaccine. A relatively new form of treatment, called Phytobiophysics, produces a range of vaccines that we have found to be equally effective in the treatment of vaccine damage. The Phytobiophysics Company has produced a kit for parents who might choose to immunise their children in this way. The company now produces a kit to immunise against the possible terrorist inspired diseases. Noni and mangosteen juices appears to effective in some case of vaccine damage. Some continental companies produce homoeopathic mixtures that have a generic potential to both immunise against viral infections and also to treat any damage that may be caused by use of orthodox injections.

So where does this leave concerned parents who are unsure what to do in the best interests of their children? Assuming that the children are fit properly nourished and with an effective immune system there appear to be five logical alternatives.

1. Do nothing and hope that if the child contracts the illness it will develop lifelong immunity without suffering any permanent damage to its health.

2. Have the injections and hope that there are no adverse effects.

3. Have the injections and to seek help at the first sign of any problems, in the knowledge that it is possible to reverse vaccine damage.

4. Have the injection and the appropriate homoeopathic vaccine at the same time. It is argued that in this way the immunisation is both effective and proof against possible vaccine

171

damage. I am aware of a colleague, still in conventional medicine, who is so concerned about the safety of the MMR. vaccine that he prefers to give the homoeopathic variety at the same time as the injection.

5. Rely entirely upon using either the homoeopathic or phyto-biophysic forms of immunisation.

I do not envy any parent having to make this decision when torn between the pressures of being told that vaccines are 100 per cent safe, not believing it, but also having to accept an alternative form of treatment that hasn't been previously personally experienced.

I have now accumulated a large numbers of newspaper clippings and Internet documents, enough to fill several books. My advice to any parent of a child who is thought to have been damaged, or indeed to any adult who believes that they have been similarly affected, to have the courage to approach their medical adviser. Since there is always a mineral deficiency demand that there is to be a full estimation of the mineral status, or at the very least for zinc, selenium and magnesium. I suspect that the request will be refused, as in a recent court case. Sooner or later a request will be granted. If there is a proven mineral deficiency that resists supplementation, but can be corrected following treatment, then the mineral deficiency theory of disease, and its treatment will be verified. It should be able to repeat similar experiments on other patients.

Postscript: April 2004 newspaper article quoting that several veterinary surgeons had written a letter claiming that multiple animal immunisations was a waste of money and amounted to fraud. Perhaps animals receive better care and support.

Chapter 22

Heredity: The Greatest Cause
For Concern

Of the six causes of disease this causes me the greatest concern. The diverse nature of this problem makes it difficult to suspect. However it could rapidly lead to an explosion in the number of ill people as it passes from one generation to another.

A colleague of mine often begins a lecture by stating that the first rule of good health is to choose one's parents wisely. This statement is guaranteed to produce a laugh, but nevertheless the parental influence is vital. The mother should be fully fit before even embarking upon pregnancy. This should include being fully stocked with minerals and vitamins, eating good wholesome food and avoiding alcohol and cigarettes. In an age where male fertility is declining, the potential father would be wise to follow the same dietary advice and lifestyle as the mother. Once conception has taken place, the father shouldn't relax and revert to smoking cigarettes because it is now known that cigarette smoke, even passively acquired, can damage the foetus leading to a possible premature birth of a small infant. The same applies to children after birth. Parental training of a child leads to the formation of lifelong habits, both good and bad, and the avoidance of the potential ill-health mine fields could well influence the length and quality of the child's life.

Despite all the best endeavours of both parents, their child may still be born with a handicap that is not immediately obvious, but eventually ill health will inevitably manifest itself after months or even years. In men this may not appear until their sixties when after a life free of illness they develop cancer. This inborn tendency is called heredity, a word that can mean different things to different people. The study of medical genetics was originally employed to unravel the mysteries of certain malformations or illnesses that appeared to be far more common in some families than others. The study was aimed at advising potential parents of

173

the percentage risks in any future pregnancies of either proceeding normally, or resulting in the birth of a palpably malformed infant. This science was then expanded to cover wider issues such as whether some families were more prone to certain forms of cancers than others. In time the study of genetic materiel yielded more clues as to the function of individual genes. This in turn led to other innovations like the cloning of animals, designer babies for whatever purpose, and the manipulation of the abnormal genes in patients with certain chronic and slowly progressive diseases. At this stage it was realised that here was another potential financial bonanza to rival pharmaceuticals and vaccines that could earn the multinational corporations vast wealth. Since then we have been bombarded with stories of how many diseases could be cured using gene therapy, or that there could be gene manipulation, or a form of vaccine to prevent certain diseases from commencing.

There have been two extreme examples trumpeted in these last few months. Firstly there is possible gene manipulation, or a vaccine to either treat or prevent cancer. This would appear to be a most laudable aim, except that some experts will state that the genetic causes of cancer are very few indeed. The two most common causes of cancer are nutritional deficiency and environmental pollution. Both these two have been covered in previous chapters, and are both amenable to simple remedies and lifestyle changes in the choice of foods, cosmetics, personal care products and household cleaners. Is this not safer and simpler than embarking upon a new and untried therapy which if it resembles its predecessors will not be free of hazards? In Chapter 19 there was a description of how in chronic viral infections, viral particles became fixed inside the nucleus of the cell and therefore possibly affecting the genes. In various testing machines this viral invasion of the nucleus can be displayed as damage to the nuclear materials RNA and DNA. Presumably even genetically modified nuclei wouldn't be immune to the attentions of viruses seeking to reproduce themselves. More recently there have been claims that certain genes have been identified that are thought to be responsible for a whole variety different conditions that includes acne. Whilst I can visualise certain stars of entertainment seeking expensive experimental treatment for their skins, and then selling their stories to various national newspapers, the rest of us should remember that acne is the result of a simple mineral deficiency, usually zinc.

The rest of this chapter will be devoted to a different concept of heredity, arising from one of the original concepts of homoeopathy. In the early days of homoeopathy correctly identified remedies worked effectively. During the course of certain epidemics, homoeopathic remedies had a better record of success than the conventional medicine of the day. In certain circumstance the same applies today. However it was found that in certain circumstance the selected remedy failed to have the desired effect. In those early years of homoeopathy there were many prevalent diseases including syphilis, cholera, typhoid, gonorrhoea, tuberculosis, the plague and many pustular conditions. It was then discovered that patients who were resistant to the obvious remedies had a strong family history where their relatives had suffered from one or other of these diseases. It was then suggested that the patient had escaped the disease that had afflicted so many relatives in the past, but had nevertheless inherited something that prevented normal homoeopathic remedies from working. So it became accepted that a homoeopathic remedy, known as a nosode, and made from infected tissue taken from other people who had a similar disease to the relatives, would be effective with, or without, the first choice of remedy.

The often-quoted example of this theory concerns children with asthma or eczema. There are several simple remedies that are normally very effective in these two conditions. When they fail to work and there is a long family history of tuberculosis, a nosode called tuberculinum is used. A homoeopath takes a full medical history, and a strong family history of tuberculosis would suggest that this particular nosode could be of use. The above theory has been brought up to date by classical homoeopaths with the notion that cancer is a modern manifestation of previous chronic illness in the family. Nosodes, made from cancerous tissues, known as carcinocins, are used for a variety of conditions, often not related to the treatment of cancer. They are amongst the most powerful and effective remedies available to medical homoeopaths. Carcinocin can also be used to treat glandular fever. Resonance homoeopathy also has a variety of remedies made up of mixtures of nosodes which can be used instead of classical remedies or where the classical remedies fail to work effectively. Unfortunately although there are occasions when this concept works, the situation is not always quite so simple.

Heredity in this context doesn't simply imply the inheriting of a disease such as cancer, or indirectly such as infantile eczema and asthma. What is inherited is the inability to absorb one or more minerals. This doesn't disprove the above theory of treatment for asthma and eczema, but merely that a child born with the inability to absorb zinc may go on to develop these two conditions or some other associated with zinc deficiency. The treatment will involve a nosode like tuberculinum. Because there is no definite or logical pattern to this inherited form of illness, only estimating the mineral levels can identify it, and then finding that taking supplements cannot rectify any deficiency. The type of machine that is used in our clinic, the Vega expert, can identify not only those minerals that are deficient and cannot easily be replenished, but it can also identify the appropriate treatment including its strength and frequency of administration. This is also why a detailed history of the health of close relatives is so important.

Therefore it is possible to inherit **any illness**; the form of the illness will be governed by which mineral or minerals aren't absorbed and the individual body's response to that deficiency. As mentioned previously it is possible to see several generations of a family, all having an identical heredity blockage to absorption, all with identical mineral deficiencies yet having entirely different illnesses. Anyone can develop the ability to pass on an inherited blockage to subsequent generations if they suffer a chronic illness before they conceive. The diseases mentioned above are not very likely to occur today, so that the most likely causes of chronic illness are parasites, viruses and vaccine damage. Candida can also cause this problem but seems less likely to do so. This is why it is so important to recognise and treat these conditions. Orthodox medicine with its emphasis on tackling symptoms, not only puts the patient at risk of side effects

176

from the drugs, but also in not treating the cause puts subsequent generations at risk, unless the patient doesn't have any children following the onset of the hereditary phenomenon. Unfortunately at the first consultation when an infective cause is found, it is often difficult to find either an inherited problem, or one that the patient has formed during the long years of undiagnosed illness. It is therefore important to review these patients several weeks following the completion of their treatment when any inherited tendency will then be more obvious.

There is usually a clue in the family history, where on one or both sides of the family there is at least one member with a chronic illness. These illnesses were mentioned in the chapter dealing with the importance of a good medical history. There are, of course, exceptions to this rule where the first person in the family chain, or an unsuspecting presumptive mother or father is symptom-less. This can happen in cases of selenium deficiency where no signs of disease have yet appeared in the family. For example, where a child is born with selenium deficiency and no signs are apparent until one day he or she is vaccinated, develops vaccine damage and only then develops symptoms. This patient will then need treatment both for the vaccine damage and the inherited damage. It is quite common to have to treat two separate conditions before a patient can fully and freely absorb all the minerals.

The treatment may be either by an appropriate nosode, or a Photobiophysic remedy. Sometimes one or two treatments will ensure a lasting cure. In other patients repeated treatments are necessary but these can have a depressing effect upon both patient and practitioner. This usually means that some vital fact has been missed. I have often found that metal toxicity from mercury fillings, or a surgical procedure can mimic heredity. If the metal toxicity is treated the apparent heredity damage disappears. This difficulty is not usually encountered when treating vaccine damage, especially when this is the only pathology present. Although I find that these two treatments are the most useful, it is possible that other treatments including high doses of powerful antioxidant mixtures, noni and mangosteen juices, some flower essences and cordyceps mushroom mixtures can work.

177

Perhaps it is now clear why this condition is so important to recognise and treat. For example take the case of a young woman with a chronic illness, such as ME. After years of this chronic illness she marries and has two children who both inherit the inability to absorb all their nutrients. Let us assume that these two children are both girls, because girls are more likely to pass on the hereditary blockage to their children (men do pass on blockages but less frequently). These two girls may or may not develop an obvious illness, but if they each have two daughters that are themselves affected, there are now possibly seven women involved. All these affected women may have either different or no symptoms. Of the seven women, six are still of an age to have further children. Since ME is quite a common condition, and there are other similar chronic diseases, it is possible to visualise a nightmare scenario where mankind is overwhelmed by a plague of different illnesses. Far-fetched vision? It does help to explain why our health services are overwhelmed, not by one disease, but by many different ones including many new ones not previously recognised. It's not too late to take decisive action, and you the reader can play your part. Any presumptive parent should ensure that the have a full complement of all minerals, vitamins, amino acids and fatty acids. There are various laboratories that can make these estimations in the event that the tests are unavailable through the NHS. If there is a full nutritional complement present in both parents, then it is most unlikely that they have any hereditary problems that can be passed to their off springs. To be 100 per cent sure then a test with a machine like the Vega expert can provide the necessary reassurance.

From a practical point of view it is just as important to review the relatives of affected patients as mentioned in the treatment of parasites. However in this case it is not the partners who are at risk but the parents, brothers, sisters and children of the patient. Many of these relatives may be symptom free, but I find that mothers are more than willing to have their children checked. If the parents or siblings are unwell then this may be the cause of their illness and the treatment is cheap, safe and effective.

I realise that this is a difficult concept to accept. However if it is not recognised and addressed then we face an explosion in the numbers of ill people. Ironically although this is potentially the greatest long-term threat to our survival, it is the cheapest and easiest to treat. All doctors could, in a very short time, gain sufficient knowledge to successfully tackle the problem

Chapter 23

Electrical Pollution Of The Environment

We have now covered five of the six basic causes of disease, namely parasites, viruses, candida, vaccination and heredity. This sixth cause of illness is perhaps the most difficult to deal with because it concerns the environment which we have grown up with and have come to accept as part of everyday life. Other environmental pollutants have been covered in previous chapters. The harmful ingredients that have been mentioned in earlier chapters can be replaced with safe products. We can choose food and drink that minimises the risk of absorbing harmful herbicides, pesticides, antibiotics, steroids, hormones or other potentially harmful ingredients. We may be at risk at work because of its hazardous nature, or exposed to chemicals in the countryside such as sheep dip. Some areas are unhealthy because of natural energies, but it is relatively easy to solve by moving away from the problem. However when it comes to a modern necessity such as electricity or a similar energy source it becomes a different matter.

To most of us, life without electricity seems unimaginable. We have learnt that electrical generation using fossil or nuclear fuels can be harmful, and there are moves towards safe renewable sources. We are also dependant upon our automobiles despite the fears of pollution and the harmful substances that are derived as by-products of the oil refining industry. How could we exist without electricity that has become such an essential part of our lives both at work and at home? The problem is that some people are very sensitive to the energy fields that surround the various conductors of electricity and the various appliances that it drives.

The problem starts with transportation of electricity from the power station to our homes and places of work. There are differing views regarding the safety of living and working too close to the overhead wires of the national grid. Some countries have planning laws that forbid the erection of buildings too near to the grid. Living in close proximity to an urban sub-station is also not without its risks. In this country we are less strict and it is possible to find even schools in close proximity to the power lines. I have seen rows of houses built directly beneath the power cables. Several studies have been conducted to see if there is a correlation between living too near to cables and developing certain cancers. So far the combined weight of governments and the electrical supply industry has been able to counter any association between these two, despite compelling evidence of such an association.

Certain odd phenomena can occur including holding an electrical fluorescent tube under power lines and watching it light up. In another example, a physicist was asked to explain the presence of a cluster of illness in a Dorset village. From the voltage of the power lines and their curvature as they descended a hill, he calculated the associated electro magnetic energy fields and found that they corresponded to the energy of a specific homoeopathic remedy that when 'overdosed' produced symptoms closely related to the cluster of illness found in the village. A Dorset GP had a practice that contained many overhead power lines. In a survey he found that the various symptoms were apparently related to the distance from the power lines where the patients lived. In another example a mother whose child suffered leukaemia decided to plot the local incidence of this childhood illness. She found that the majority lived close to power lines and sub-stations, and there also appeared to be a correlation between living in a cul-de-sac or near a water supply end main. Unfortunately all her research, which was placed upon the computer system of a Medical Officer for Health was somehow 'lost'. The woman who compiled this information also lost her husband to cancer, and they had lived in close proximity to pylons. In addition she noted that a perfectly normal neighbour would suddenly appear and sweep her drive and behave in a very odd manner whenever it rained. There are now scientists who specialise in the study of electrical and electro-magnetic fields that are formed in close proximity to the national grid, and their research is ongoing. Here is another example where some of our continental neighbours acknowledge this problem and have developed machines to test for it and treatments to deal with it. There will be other examples in this chapter where the

Government and the industry will continue to claim that power supply is 100 per cent safe, but an increasing number of people are beginning to have their doubts.

We certainly find a small number of people who are adversely affected by electrically powered appliances. Many people who live in the area of our clinic work in call centres where they are surrounded by of a multitude of computers, telephones and other electrical appliances in addition to miles of electrical cables. Obviously not all the employees are affected, but there are examples of 'sick building syndrome'. It is not obvious why some people are affected and others aren't, but it is possible that some other underlying condition makes them more susceptible than their work colleagues. Our homes are crammed with electrical appliances. A favourite to cause trouble is the electric blanket, especially when it is left switched on all night. The bedroom is a particularly dangerous place because we spend a significant amount of time there, and lying roughly in the same position. In general there is a direct correlation between any unhealthy influence and the time spent subject to it. Electrical appliances in their bedrooms often surround children and it is not uncommon to find an electric blanket, teasmade/alarm, computer, Hi-Fi and TV.

Downstairs is not much safer with all the electrical appliances that generate a multitude of electro-magnetic fields. Lastly in the kitchen there is the ever-present microwave machine, an essential in today's hectic life. Microwaves are dangerous, and a machine that leaks is especially so. Few people have their machine checked to see if it leaks. However there is a more sinister reason to be wary of microwaves. Kerlian photography shows that food cooked in a microwave is completely denatured. The importance of nutrition, or rather the lack of it, is vitally important in the maintenance of good health. The Russian Government banned microwaves but had to relax the laws because of pressure from the vested commercial interests of the post communist era. Once again, we see human health compromised in favour of such vested interests.

Another microwave appliance to make the headlines is the mobile phone, to which many people, including young children, have become addicted, despite repeated evidence that these appliances can be harmful. Research has shown that the relative thinness of a child's skull makes it more prone to damage from the microwave emissions of mobile phones. The British Government has made a very half-hearted attempt to warn children and their parents of these dangers. However another Government department complained that such warnings were harming the industry. I suppose that this is not surprising since the various companies were almost bankrupted by the high fees paid to our Government for their operating licenses. Again health has been compromised. Various attachments have been made in an attempt to reduce the resulting radiation reaching the brain. The manufacturers say that this is unnecessary, but surprisingly they have carried out their own research with a view to installing their own protective devices, 'to put the minds of people at rest'. Whoever heard of companies spending unnecessary money on unessential products to alleviate the concerns of the public? Why do people study the tables of the emissions from the various different makes of mobile telephone? There have been several reports of brain cancer associated with the prolonged use of mobile phones. A local consultant noted an apparent increase in the number of unilateral brain tumours, but didn't appear to have enquired about the use of mobile phones and which ear was used. Certainly we have seen examples of cancer and other conditions in close proximity to where switched on phones are kept close to the body, either tucked into the belt or trouser back pocket. Impaired memory, constant headache and migraine are frequently associated with persistent use of mobile phones. The use of earpieces offers no protection and, the only reliable protection is from an all over shield for the phone. If there is any doubt about the effect of transmissions of radio or microwaves there is the story of a house situated between two transmission bowls at G.C.H.Q. where the television sets had a habit of exploding. In the USA scientists are reportedly working upon a microwave weapon that is reportedly very powerful. In a separate development the use of microwaves to destroy breast cancer cells is being investigated

It is possible to argue that the use of mobile phones and any personal damage that they may cause is a matter of personal choice. However like the problem of cigarette smoking it is not quite so simple. It seems that using a mobile phone within a rigid cage like a train carriage causes an increased intensity of induced radiation as the emissions from the phones bounce off the metal walls. Perhaps there could be an increase in taxation to cover the additional cost of illness. However life is not so simple because mobile phones need mobile phone masts and they too pose a health risk for those people living nearby. Once again Government and the telephone industry rush to tell us that they pose no threat to health. Certainly we frequently come across people who are unwell until they move away from a mobile phone mast. The problem can be accentuated if a person lives between two or three masts. Government has tried to stop local councils refusing planning applications to erect masts purely on the grounds of a danger to health. There are however several court cases pending, where people are challenging the law that doesn't permit objections to phone masts on the grounds of safety. Despite the claims that these masts are safe the companies go to great lengths to disguise them as trees or buried inside church steeples or petrol station signs. They pay schools, churches and other organisations to have them on their premises, and the authorities would prefer to accept the payment rather than show concern for the children and parishioners. In other circumstances they affix the antennae to existing poles. We have examples of people becoming ill and being unaware that antennae had been erected overnight. However evidence is accumulating of the harmful effects upon the health that these technologies pose. Recently an influential group of German doctors have been persuaded that the dangers to health are very real and published an article stating their views. The Swiss Government has licensed a product to protect people against a variety of radiations. We have tried both the mobile version and the larger module to protect a whole house, and they both would appear to be successful. There are also homoeopathic remedies and ornaments containing imploded water that can undo, or even protect against, the harmful effects of radiations.

Articles in the press frequently quote the perceived dangers of microwave appliances, especially the telephones and masts. These and other dangers to our society appear almost daily. The press fail to pursue the issues in the same way that they champion other causes. How long will we have to wait before the public takes action to force governments to protect them from the dangers to our collective health?

Electricity is not the only pollutant to affect our health. However the effects of other pollutants have been covered in previous chapters.

Postscript

Not The End: Just The Beginning

Between them Hitler and Stalin have been credited with the slaughter of many millions of people. Following the Second World War, slaughter on such a grand scale has moved from Europe to Africa. On the African continent a series of civil wars have resulted in the death of countless people either through genocide or by wilful and preventable starvation. In the Western democracies we pride ourselves that slaughter on such a massive scale has now been consigned to history, and therefore couldn't happen here again. However such complacency begs two questions. Firstly why haven't we intervened in the African civil wars that have dragged on for so very many years? It would appear that we have stood idly by and only occasionally satisfying our consciences with the provision of aid relief. In other parts of the world the Western democracies have intervened with the flimsiest of pretexts if their own perceived national interests were threatened. Secondly why, throughout the world, have we permitted countless numbers of people to fall victim of preventable and even treatable diseases? Nobody can deny the relentless increase in cancer, heart and other chronic illnesses, including the AIDS epidemic in Africa. Patients are left with lifelong chronic debilitating illness, or they are consigned to an early and painful death, often accelerated by the medical treatment that they have received.

Is it possible that our so-called democracies have condoned and contributed to the ill health and death of so many members of our societies? Is there a hidden agenda to seek a reduction in the world population, not by war, but by new and subtler means? Would various governments conceive and sanction such methods designed to reduce populations? Such schemes to reduce populations would demand concerted action by many governments and therefore there would need to be a coordinating body. It seems most unlikely that individual governments would pursue such identical policies that had been spontaneously arrived at without

186

any prior knowledge of the intentions of other administrations. Could our leaders permit an outside organisation to dictate to them what legislation to enact? According to various sources even the apparently powerful American Presidents are covertly influenced by outside bodies. This may explain the financial connection between the members of the American Administration, both elected and appointed, and major industrial conglomerates.

Another example of concerted action from closer to home could have a detrimental effect upon whole populations. Member Governments of the European Union are in the process of banning, or restricting, the sale of various minerals and vitamins. In this book and in countless other medical publications there are examples of how the deficiency of nutrients can lead to disease. For nearly seventy years it has been known that farm produce is inherently deficient in nutrition. These proposed restrictions on the sale of nutrients will inevitably lead to increases in chronic illness and death. The drug companies and governments appear to be the sole financial beneficiaries of such actions. Perhaps it offers an explanation as to why the authorities consistently resist attempts to estimate the nutritional status of patients. If universal estimation of nutrients were permitted then the European Directive would be seen to be against the best interests of patients, and it could destroy the very credibility of the European Union.

Who are these supreme powerful organisations? Certainly the vast wealth of certain global industries that includes various chemical, petrochemical and pharmaceutical conglomerates could be involved. International banks and financial institutions have sufficient wealth to enable them to wield powerful influences for both good and evil. In concert these industries and financial institutions are capable of directly influencing both election of and the performance of governments. However they are more likely to exert their power and influence through other agencies. Not unnaturally a variety of names and organisations have been accused of being the worldwide power brokers. America is a rich source of many of these theories. Under the various freedom of information acts Americans are allowed to scrutinise their Government's documents. Some of these documents that have been released after the statutory time delay, detail the financial involvement and support for Hitler and the holocaust by various financial organisations and political dynasties. These same families and organisations are still prominent in current American society, being involved in both politics and industry. This influence extends to the control and funding of hospitals and medical research.

The possibility that there is a supreme body that orchestrates world events seems plausible. The alternative assumption is that many Governments are ill informed or even ignorant about the slide into ill health and a consequent reduction in the population of the world. How else could the events described in this book occur without at the very least the cooperation of Governments?

The practice of medicine is dominated by the drug industry from the moment a student enters medical school and throughout the years in practice right up to the moment of retirement. Although doctors might seek be absolved from any blame, nevertheless they should have realised that the present practice of medicine is failing to deliver any general improvement in health In fact the reverse is true with the rapid increase in all forms of chronic disease. Doctors have, with possible exception of tobacco, stood idly by and chosen to ignore the many other harmful threats to health. Why have they neglected to warn patients about the many toxic chemicals in our environment, including some in the very medicines that they themselves prescribe? Why have they supported the addition of toxic fluoride to our water when other countries have abandoned it because of the failure to reduce dental decay? Fluoride is both carcinogenic and can render bones brittle? If for no other reason they should have opposed fluoridisation on the grounds of mass medication with no upper safe limit on the total dosage of the chemical taken into the body. Medical authorities have also joined with their dental colleagues in declaring that the mercury in dental amalgam is harmless. Why are doctors become involved in one of the biggest medical frauds by prescribing HRT when very few women are deficient in oestrogen and progesterone? Is it possible that after thousands of years women have suddenly

188

become deficient in oestrogen in the menopausal years? Why should HRT prevent many other diseases like heart disease, strokes, cancer and osteoporosis? Women who have been healthy and given birth to one or more children already have sufficient stores of progesterone in their bodies and therefore do not need additional, and synthetic hormones. These women usually have sufficient oestrogen because the body continues to produce this hormone after the menopause. In addition it is almost impossible to avoid taking in the additional oestrogens that can be found in water and various foods. For women with any hormone deficiency it is usually the result of a mineral deficiency. Mineral deficiency and not hormone deficiency is often the cause of osteoporosis. Why give extra oestrogen when it can increase the risk of cancer? Why recommend dairy when it can make osteoporosis worse? Why believe that testosterone causes prostate cancer? Can antibiotics be safe? The biggest question of all is why do professionals selected and trained to be observant and with enquiring minds accept all this without the slightest hesitation? Doctors may have received little or no training in nutrition, but they are capable of their own research into the many available textbooks and articles on this subject. Many doctors must have been asked for dietary advice by patients who themselves have read worrying articles in both newspapers and magazines.

Did anyone complain when tobacco and certain drugs pronounced too toxic for use in the Western democracies were actively marketed in the Third World? It is no wonder that those people who are interested in ethical banking and investment find great difficulty in finding a home for their money. Do we honestly believe that all the research and development will lead to the cure of serious illness when such treatment would damage the financial health of those same industries? Can we really wait for another fifty years to find a cure for cancer? There have been several inventions that have been bought out by rival companies simply to prevent a potential competitor reaching the market place. Scientists have been threatened with the withdrawal of their grants if the results of their research conflicts with the interests of the sponsor. This then casts doubt over all forms of medical research especially when allegedly supporting a particular drug or treatment. Only positive news is tolerated, and it must not be forgotten that drug companies sponsor nearly all drug research in hospitals.

None of these facts are hidden. There are almost daily exposures in the media. Despite this no newspaper, magazine of broadcast organisation seems willing to pursue these issues, presumably because they fear losing advertising revenue. In America the general public seems more aware of the facts, but chooses to accept the corruptness of the system. In Great Britain we are certainly becoming better informed, but I hope that we don't follow the American example of tacit toleration. Can we honestly believe, without exception, that Government is committed to improving our health?

So why is so much money spent upon the research and development of new chemicals? The same money would be better spent on determining the toxicity or otherwise of the thousands of new chemicals that have been created and released into our environment. However the money required to prove or refute a nutritional theory of disease/health would be miniscule in comparison with the drug companies' research funds. Hospital laboratories routinely estimate the blood content of only a few selected minerals. These minerals are often affected as a consequence of medical treatment. Therefore if the technology exists why do laboratories continue to refuse to estimate minerals like selenium, magnesium, zinc and chromium whose deficiencies are responsible for the majority of all chronic illnesses? The refusal to make these blood estimations can only mean that the consequences of mineral deficiencies are well known and that any additional confirmation and publication would not be in the best interests of the drug companies and therefore cannot be tolerated. I consider that there can be no other explanation for the refusal to make available these blood tests. Billions of pounds are spent annually in an attempt to cope with an ever-increasing volume of ill health. Surely a concerned Government would spend a miniscule amount from the health budget to carry out some simple research to verify the concept of disease as outlined in this book. Such simple research could prove, or disprove, the safety of vaccines. If Government is so confident about the safety of its immunisation programme it would spend this small amount of money. A positive result from this research would be cheaper and more persuasive than its current propaganda designed to reassure anxious parents. Government must know that an increasing number of people distrust any official statement, and therefore I am left to assume that they are either extremely arrogant or that they are party to a predetermined plan that is designed to increase the levels of ill health and as a result reduce the size of the population, especially the elderly and more expensive sections of society.

It would seem that the origins of disease are either unknown or deliberately ignored for selfish financial reasons. As a consequence of this the majority of statistical research into the effectiveness of modern treatments is flawed. For example it is erroneously accepted that osteoporosis is the result of a deficiency in oestrogen and/or calcium. Progesterone (the natural variety) magnesium and boron deficiencies are ignored. The reality is that there is often too much oestrogen and a deficiency of one or more of progesterone, magnesium and boron. Of the three the two minerals are the most common causes of osteoporosis. If there is a failure to measure the two minerals what valid reason is there for comparing synthetic with natural hormone therapies in the treatment of osteoporosis? Equally how is it possible to compare any synthetic and natural product? Scientists must be aware of the consequences of mineral and vitamin deficiencies. They must also be aware of the deficiencies in food. Their masters must be equally aware of these facts and therefore it must be assumed there is a deliberate policy to suppress such information that could only lead to an increase in health and a decrease in company profits. The only logical explanation is that there is a worldwide conspiracy to perpetuate disease and to selectively reduce the world population.

No effort is spared in trying to rubbish the claims made for nutritional products and the various alternative therapies. These attacks appear to be orchestrated by the drug companies themselves, whilst at the same time they are purchasing many companies and clinics associated with these therapies. No expense is spared in the attempts to rubbish any attacks on their own pharmaceutical products. Hence recent newspaper headlines such as "HRT what are women to believe?"

Is there any hope for society? There is a wealth of knowledge available, especially on the Internet. It is relatively easy for anyone to carry out his or her own research. If anyone decides to carry their own experiment then there a number of private laboratories that will carry out requests for specified mineral estimations. I am confident that a relatively inexpensive research project will demonstrate that vaccines can damage health. In addition relatively small investments can demonstrate that treatment can restore the ability of the body to absorb minerals. People must take responsibility for their own health and assume that they alone have their best interests at heart.

It is possible that by self-help we can learn how to stay healthy, and should it become necessary how also to regain health. When sufficient numbers of people take the responsibility for their own health there will be an unstoppable movement to weaken the present influence exerted by governments. At the same time we can weaken the power of certain sinister organisations that have exerted undue influence over those people that we have elected to protect us. Perhaps issues such as the fluoridisation of water or the restriction of minerals and vitamins will awaken members of the public to the dangers of the Government's policies.

This book reveals how simple it is to understand the issues surrounding both health and ill health. There are six easily identified and treatable basic causes of disease. These are parasites, viruses, candida, vaccines, heredity and environmental pollutants. Treatments can be cheap safe and effective. Many pharmaceutical products could work if correctly chosen. Underpinning all this is the correct lifestyle and the correct use of supplements, both for treatment and prevention. It is not rocket science and any one can achieve good health. Why cannot doctors do it?

We are left with the inescapable conclusion that there is a worldwide conspiracy of governments and large corporations to maintain, or even increase, the incidence of disease and premature death. The only question that remains is the degree to which the medical profession is involved in this conspiracy. In their defence it could be argued that all their education is controlled by organisations that have a vested interest in the maintenance of high levels of disease. Also as a consequence of this failure to control disease doctors are kept so busy that there is a very little time left for reflection and individual research. So the final question remains to be answered. Is there evidence of **treason within our society and who is involved?**

Appendix A

Sodium Lauryl Sulphate

1. Improper eye development in children. Affects protein structures and keeps children's eyes from developing properly.
2. Can cause cataracts.
3. Proven skin irritant.
4. Penetrates into heart, brain, liver etc.
5. If contaminated with certain chemicals can form carcinogenic chemicals that are easily absorbed into the body.

Propylene Glycol

1. Breathing of mist can irritate nose and chest.
2. Swallowing can cause nausea, vomiting and diarrhoea.
3. In laboratory animals causes liver and kidney damage.
4. First aid:
   If on skin wash thoroughly with soap and water. Remove contaminated clothing.
   If in eyes, flush out with large amounts of water.
   If swallowed immediately drink two glasses of water and induce vomiting.
   If breathed, remove to fresh air.
   Primary route of damage via the skin.

Appendix B

Some of the potentially harmful ingredients commonly used by the personal care industry.

Alcohol
Alpha H
Alpha Hydroxy Acid
Alcohol
Animal fat
Bentonite
Collagen
Dioxins
Elastin of high-molecular weight
Fluorocarbons
Formaldehyde
Glycerin
Kaolin
Lanolin
Lye
Mineral oil
Petrolatum
Sodium laureth sulphate
Talc

Appendix C

Some of the diseases caused by deficiencies due to the most important 6 minerals.

BORON
Defective hormone function
Interferes with proper use of calcium and magnesium
Poor bone metabolism and cause of osteoporosis
Defective hormone function

CHROMIUM
ADD/ADHD
Anxiety
Blood sugar disturbance
Cholesterol and heart disease
Fatigue
Hyperactivity
Learning difficulties
Rages

LITHIUM
ADD
Depression
Manic depression
Rages and fits

MAGNESIUM
Anxiety
Anorexia
Confusion
Depression
Constipation
High and low blood pressure
Hyperactivity
Insomnia
Irritability

ME

Menstrual pains cramps and migraines
Muscle pains, cramps and twitches
Neuromuscular problems
Osteoporosis
Palpitations
Vertigo

SELENIUM

'Age' spots
Alzheimer's disease and any memory problems
Cancer
Cataracts
Cot death
Fatigue
Heart disease and palpitations
Hormonal problems due to effect upon the pituitary gland
Hyperactivity and various educational diseases including autism
Liver cirrhosis
Multiple sclerosis, muscular dystrophy and Parkinson's disease
Pancreatitis
Poor Immunity
Severe pain with often no apparent cause
Scoliosis (twisted spine)
Susceptibility to vaccine damage

ZINC

Acne
Allergies
Anaemia
Asthma
Apathy, depression and irritability
Eczema
Fatigue
Loss of taste and smell
Nails that are brittle and have white spots.
Poor wound healing
Poor immunity with frequent colds

Appendix D

Lack of essential fatty acids may cause

ADD/ADHD and hyperactivity
Allergies
Asthma
Brittle nails
Dry skin and hair
Dandruff
Eczema
Excessive and hard ear wax
Excessive thirst
Multiple sclerosis and similar diseases
Poor attention span
Premenstrual tension

Appendix E

Some vaccines can contain:

Aluminium
Animal tissue (pig, horse, rabbit, dog monkey chicken, sheep and calf)
Antibiotics
Colourants
Ethylene glycol
Formaldehyde
Formalin
Gelatin
Human foetal cells
Monosodium glutamate
Mercury
Sugars
Various other antiseptics and preservatives